Sports Gynecology: Problems and Care of the Athletic Female

Sports Gynecology: Problems and Care of the Athletic Female

Michelle P. Warren, MD
Professor of Obstetrics
  and Gynecology and Medicine
  Columbia College of Physicians
  and Surgeons;
Co-Director, Reproductive Endocrinology
Medical Director, Women's Center for Health and Social Issues
St. Luke's/Roosevelt Hospital
New York, New York

Mona M. Shangold, MD
Director, Center for Sports Gynecology and
  Women's Health
Philadelphia, Pennsylvania

b

**Blackwell
Science**

2000

AUG

Blackwell Science
Editorial offices:
238 Main Street, Cambridge,
  Massachusetts 02142, USA
Osney Mead, Oxford OX2 0El, England
25 John Street, London WC1N 2BL,
  England
23 Ainslie Place, Edinburgh EH3 6AJ,
  Scotland
54 University Street, Carlton, Victoria
  3053, Australia
Other Editorial Offices:
Arnette Blackwell SA, 224, Boulevard
  Saint Germain, 75007 Paris, France
Blackwell Wissenschafts-Verlag GmbH
  Kurfürstendamm 57, 10707 Berlin,
  Germany
Zehetnergasse 6, A-1140 Vienna, Austria

Distributors:
USA
  Blackwell Science, Inc.
  238 Main Street
  Cambridge, Massachusetts 02142
  (Telephone orders: 800-215-1000
  or 617-876-7000;
  Fax orders: 617-492-5263)

Canada
  Copp Clark Professional
  200 Adelaide Street, West, 3rd Floor
  Toronto, Ontario M5H 1W7
  Telephone orders: 416-597-1616
  1-800-815-9417; fax: 416-597-1617

Australia
  Blackwell Science Pty., Ltd.
  54 University Street
  Carlton, Victoria 3053
  (Telephone orders: 03-9347-0300;
  fax: 03-9349 3016)

Outside North America and Australia
  Blackwell Science, Ltd.
  c/o Marston Book Services, Ltd.
  P.O. Box 269
  Abingdon
  Oxon OX14 4YN
  England
  (Telephone orders: 44-01235-465500;
  fax: 44-01235-465555)

Acquisitions: Jim Krosschell
Production: Heather Garrison
Manufacturing: Lisa Flanagan
Typeset by Best-set Typesetter Ltd.
Printed and bound by Edwards Brothers

©1997 by Blackwell Science, Inc.

Printed in the United States of America

96 97 98 99 5 4 3 2 1

The Blackwell Science logo is a trade mark
of Blackwell Science Ltd., registered at the
United Kingdom Trade Marks Registry

Library of Congress Cataloging-in-
Publication Data

Warren, Michelle P.
    Sports gynecology / Michelle P.
Warren, Mona Shangold.
      p. cm.
    Includes bibliographical references
and index.
    ISBN 0-86542-463-2
    1. Sports gynecology. I. Shangold,
Mona M. II. Title.
    [DNLM: 1. Gynecology.
2. Women's Health. 3. Sports.
WP 100
W291s 1996]
RG207.W37 1996
618.1—dc21
DNLM/DLC
for Library of Congress   96-48787
                                      CIP

To my (M. W.) husband, Fiske
  our sons, Matthew and Christopher Warren, and Kenny Mirkin,
  and my (M. S.) father, Jack Shangold.

In memory of my (M. W.) father, Edmund L. Palmieri
  and our mothers, Claude Verron Palmieri and Harriet Shangold.

And to the many patients and athletes who have inspired us and taught us
  so much.

Contents

Preface

Women have become increasingly physically active in the past several decades. As a result, there is an urgent need for practical information about the obstetric and gynecologic care of exercising women. This book is intended for physicians and other persons, including health care providers, trainers and coaches, who take care of women who exercise. We review all the common issues relative to gynecologic and reproductive problems. Since the problems women face can vary greatly depending on their age and hormonal status, this book also presents a review of the normal physiology. This is important because minor deviations from normal can occur in competitive situations. This can be upsetting to the athletes even though these deviations are of minor medical significance. The common problems are also divided according to age and hormonal status. Puberty and menopause have been given special emphasis— puberty, because it is a vulnerable time, and menopause, because with an aging population more women are exercising. This book also attempts to answer some of the important questions asked by women concerning such topics as the effects of exercise on pregnancy and, in the case of serious athletes, the effects of the menstrual cycle and hormones on training and performance. Lastly, the overwhelming positive effects of exercise are reviewed, as are some of the commonly abused performance enhancers.

Whenever possible, we have presented the scientific background in support of our advice. However, in many cases, scientific studies have not yet answered all the questions we face in caring for exercising women. For those problems lacking controlled studies, we have presented rational plans that are based on current knowledge and our own experience, derived from years of clinical practice, for advising and managing patients. We have been careful to distinguish between the advice supported by science and that supported by our experience.

We hope this book provides practical information to health care providers, coaches, trainers, and athletes, and we hope it inspires researchers to provide even more answers to questions in the growing field of sports gynecology.

Acknowledgements

Particularly deserving of recognition are Ms. Eliza Geer and Ms. Lisa Golomb, who researched and collaborated with the authors on several chapters The Adult Athlete: Performance Enhancing Drugs, The Adult Athlete: Gynecologic Problems and Performance (EG); The Adult Athlete: Dysmenorrhea, The Adult Athlete: Premenstrual Syndrome, The Adult Athlete: Other Gynecologic Problems, and The Adult Athlete: Complications of Reproductive Problems (LG). They have moved on to medical school and careers where they will continue to apply their writing talents.

M.P.W.
M.M.S.

CHAPTER

1

The Female Athlete

The Female and Sports

The number of women and girls exercising on a regular basis has grown greatly during the past 30 years, and physicians now have more female patients engaging in regular exercise programs than ever before. Long-distance runners who run more than 70 miles per week are not unusual in the 1990s. The only woman who ran in the 1970 New York City Marathon did not finish; 20 years later, in 1990, 5249 women entered and 4500 finished. Physicians must be prepared to advise the ever increasing number of patients about the risks and benefits of exercise and manage any problems that arise along the way.

Why More Women Are Exercising Now

Many factors have contributed to the increased physical activity of women, including research demonstrating exercise benefits, media dissemination of such information, legislation creating more opportunities, implementation of such laws, cultural changes permitting and encouraging women to become more active, and physician endorsement and advocacy of such efforts. Each of these factors alone would have increased the number of women participating in exercise programs. Collectively, these factors have led to an exponential rise in the numbers and percentages of women exercising.

Scientific Research Many years ago, female athletes were rare and often were treated by society with disrespect and nonacceptance. Young girls were socially programmed at an early age to avoid exercise, which was

1

deemed "unfeminine" and inappropriate. Scientific researchers gave female exercisers little attention, and, as a result, little was known about the effects of exercise upon women and girls. Their entry into the ranks of both serious and casual athletes permitted and encouraged scientific research, which led to the surprising findings that 1) exercise is beneficial for women, and 2) exercise may help to prevent and treat several diseases prevalent among women.

Media Endorsement and Exposure   The media were quick to propagate these findings to the public, and many previously sedentary women realized that exercise is important for everyone. Lay literature about the benefits of exercise became abundant, and women found that they could achieve many personal goals by developing and following a program of regular physical exercise. The entry of numerous celebrities into the exercise movement helped convince those who remained skeptical of exercise benefits, particularly when it ran so contrary to the principles upon which they were raised.

Legislation   The passage of Title IX of the Educational Amendment Act of 1972 mandated that women and girls must have opportunities equal to those of men and boys in physical education and athletics in all educational institutions receiving federal funds. The subsequent implementation of this legislative amendment provided new opportunities for women in both competitive and casual athletics. This served to encourage even more women and girls to exercise regularly.

Cultural Changes   Although it had been common in certain ethnic cultures long ago for women to be physically active, this was not the case in the United States prior to 1972, when Title IX legislation was passed. Cultural changes since then have led to a much greater acceptance of women athletes, as well as an alteration in the image of the ideal woman from one who is slender and devoid of both muscle and fat to one who is lean and muscular. The former ideal woman depended on cigarettes to achieve her image, whereas the newer ideal woman is much more likely to use exercise. The many celebrities who have revealed their vigorous exercise habits have encouraged their fans to develop a regular exercise routine. Women want to believe that they can look like Jane Fonda if they exercise enough, even if it isn't true.

Physician Endorsement   The role of supportive physicians cannot be over-stated, because many women turn to their physicians for advice about health and fitness. Until physicians became regular exercisers themselves, women found it difficult to convince themselves that exercise is beneficial for everyone. ("If my physician doesn't think it's important to exercise, why should I?") Physicians and other health care providers had to serve as both educators and role models in order to accomplish this. They had to first learn the benefits of regular exercise, then learn to incorporate physical activity into their own lives, and finally convince their female patients that exercise is worth the time and effort.

Categorization of Women by Exercise Habits and Goals

In order to convince and encourage women to exercise, health care providers must be familiar with all the benefits of regular exercise and must be able to relate these favorable consequences to individual patients with unique goals, interests, and impediments. Women tend to fall into three major categories, based on their exercise habits and motivations: 1) serious athletes who train because they enjoy the experience of the sport, 2) regular exercisers who train because they believe it helps them to achieve an important goal (cardiovascular fitness, weight loss, and so on), and 3) sedentary women who have not yet been convinced that exercise is worth the time and effort required. Health care providers must be aware of each patient's category in order to provide each with optimal advice.

Why Women Exercise Regularly

Regular exercise can help women achieve many goals, and women differ in the goals they consider important. Among the many benefits of regular exercise and training, the following can serve as realistic goals for any woman: enhanced cardiovascular fitness, improved physical endurance and work capacity, greater muscle mass and strength, increased bone density, reduced adiposity, improved physical appearance, greater flexibility, improved neuromuscular coordination, improved cognitive function, improved affect, improved sleep quality, and, as a result of many of these improvements, improved quality of life, particularly among those for whom weakness imposed obvious limitations on self-sufficiency.

These goals can be used to encourage sedentary women to start a regular exercise habit. Those who are already exercising on a regular basis probably do so for some of these reasons. Competitive and other serious athletes may have as additional goals the improvements in speed, strength, and neuromuscular coordination that are necessary components of athletic success.

Encouraging Women to Exercise

Successful programs aimed at encouraging regular participation in sports must determine the specific goals that are important to each woman and must be tailored to each woman as an individual. To attract and keep women as regular exercisers, such programs must first overcome the negative attitudes many women have toward exercise and must ensure that they undertake programs that will help them achieve realistic goals. Those who are already exercising regularly must continue to achieve their goals if they are expected to keep exercising.

Competitive athletes also need encouragement and support from physicians. They must receive current and accurate information from their physicians about training, competition, and medical problems. If their medical conditions affect or are affected by exercise or training, they must be advised honestly about all treatment options. They must be informed about whether continued training will affect the disease or its treatment, and whether the disease and its treatment will have any effect upon exercise or training.

Special Problems of Different Athletic Disciplines
Genetic Issues

The female athlete derives many benefits from exercise but is also at special risk because of the sensitivity of the reproductive system to environmental stresses. At the same time, the somatotype of the individual may be a determining factor in the choice of an athletic discipline, and some women may be socialized into a particular sport because their physique puts them at a competitive advantage. These physical attributes, which are genetically determined, may also be associated with genetic tendencies to menstrual dysfunction. It is often difficult to separate the environmental influences from the genetic; both should be considered in evaluating the female athlete. Retrospective studies of swimmers and gymnasts have shown that differences in height (swimmers are taller than average and gymnasts shorter) are apparent at 3 years of age.

Environmental Issues

Stress   One of the most obvious environmental influences is the level of stress associated with the athletic discipline. Some sports are much more rigorous in terms of training hours and competitive demands. Another important factor is the intensity at which the elite athlete competes at a national or international level. Some activities, such as figure skating, gymnastics, and ballet, require training at a very young age, when the reproductive system is immature and much more vulnerable to both psychological and physical stress.

Physical Stress   Some disciplines—such as long-distance running, ballet, figure skating, and gymnastics—require low body weight for optimal performance; others—such as swimming—put more emphasis on strength than on weight.

Low Body Weight   The emphasis on body weight may be a factor, however, even when performance is not the main issue, because appearance may be part of the scoring process in such sports as diving, figure skating, and gymnastics. Close-fitting clothing worn in an athletic event may emphasize body shape, and a slender line may bring higher scores. Other sports, such as rowing, require weight categories, thus emphasizing weight in less subtle ways.

Performance Enhancers   A more recent problem for the female athlete is the use of performance-enhancing drugs, such as anabolic steroids and growth hormone. Although these drugs are used mainly to improve strength, they may have a profound effect on the reproductive system as well as on the skin and voice. These drugs are more apt to be used in sports that emphasize strength for performance, such as track and swimming.

Organ Systems at Risk in the Female Athlete   Athletic training may have a direct effect on the female reproductive organs or an indirect effect on the delicate signals to the hypothalamic pituitary ovarian axis. Some effects may be positive, such as alleviation of dysmenorrhea, while others may be worrisome, such as irregular periods or bladder incontinence due to pressure of the pelvic organs on the urinary tract. Menstrual dysfunction has been found in many athletic disciplines; recent evidence indicates that a group of such problems are due to low body weight or a so-called energy drain, in which the caloric intake is insufficient to maintain the athlete's level of activity. The incidence of menstrual problems in different athletic disciplines is shown in Table 1.1. Eating disorders may be common in these groups, the epidemiology and hormonal profile of which have been well characterized.

Recent evidence has found another type of amenorrhea, described in swimmers, that is characterized by mild hyperandrogenism and is either genetically determined or secondary to intensive training and activation of the adrenal axis (see Figure 1.1).

Table 1.1 *Surveys of the prevalence of amenorrhea and oligomenorrhea in different athletic disciplines*

Activity	Study	n	Percentage with Irregularities
General population	Petterson et al (1973)	1862	1.8
	Singh (1981)	900	5.0
Weight-bearing sports			
Ballet	Abraham et al (1982)	29	79.0
	Brooks-Gunn et al (1987)	53	59.0
	Feicht et al (1978)	128	6–43
	Glass et al (1987)	67	34.0
Running	Shangold and Levine (1982)	394	24.0
	Sanborn et al (1982)	237	26.0
Non-weight-bearing sports			
Cycling	Sanborn et al (1982)	33	12.0
Swimming	Sanborn et al (1982)	197	12.0

Reproduced by permission from Constantini NW, Warren MP. Physical activity, fitness and reproductive health in women. In: Bouchard C, Shephard RJ, Stephens T, eds. Physical activity, fitness and health 1992 proceedings, Champaign, IL: Human Kinetics Publishers, 1994:955–966, p. 957.

Hypothesis: Menstrual Dysfunction In Different Types of Sports

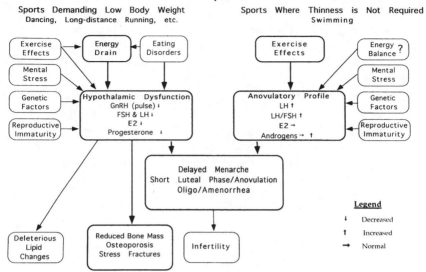

Figure 1.1 *A hypothesis of two different mechanisms leading to athletes' menstrual dysfunction. The first (left side) is seen in sports demanding very low weight and results in hypothalamic dysfunction and prolonged periods of hypoestrogenism with the serious consequence of osteoporosis. The second (right side) suggests a different mechanism that might exist in sports that do not require thinness, such as swimming. (Reproduced by permission from Constantini NW, Warren MP. Physical activity, fitness and reproductive health in women. In: Bouchard C, Shephard RJ, Stephens T, eds. Physical activity, fitness and health 1992 proceedings, Champaign, IL: Human Kinetics, 1994:955–966, p. 960.)*

Finally, the female athlete may put herself at risk by the use of the so-called performance-enhancing drugs, all of which have multiple effects on different organ systems. Furthermore, they affect the young adolescent girl differently from the mature adult.

Bibliography

1. Abraham SF, Beumont PJV, Fraser IS, et al. Body weight, exercise and menstrual status among ballet dancers in training. Br J Obstet Gynaecol 1982;89:507–510.

2. Brooks-Gunn J, Burrow C, Warren MP. Attitudes toward eating and body weight in different groups of female adolescent athletes. Int J Eat Disord 1988;7(6):749–757.
3. Feicht CB, Johnson TS, Martin BJ, et al. Secondary amenorrhea in athletes. Lancet 1978;2:1145–1146.
4. Glass AR, Deuster PA, Kyle SB, et al. Amenorrhea in Olympic marathon runners. Fertil Steril 1987;48:740–745.
5. Petterson F, Fries H, Nillius SJ. Epidemiology of secondary amenorrhea: incidence and prevalence rates. Am J Obstet Gynecol 1973;7:80–86.
6. Sanborn CF, Martin BJ, Wagner WW, Jr. Is athletic amenorrhea specific to runners? Am J Obstet Gynecol 1982;143:859–861.
7. Shangold MM, Levine HS. The effect of marathon training upon menstrual function. Am J Obstet Gynecol 1982;143:862–869.
8. Singh KB. Menstrual disorders in college students. Am J Obstet Gynecol 1981;1210:299–302.

CHAPTER
2

Normal Puberty and Menarche

Initiation of Puberty

The Hypothalamic Pituitary Axis

The event that initiates puberty is the activation of the secretion of gonadotropin releasing hormone (GnRH) in an area of the brain called the hypothalamus. This hormone is initially secreted at night and then over a 24-hour period in rhythmic spurts occurring every 60 to 90 minutes. This rhythm is controlled by the pulse generator, which is situated in the arcuate nucleus in the medial central area of the hypothalamus. The net effect of these changes is to activate the hypothalamic pituitary ovarian axis: GnRH stimulates the gonadotropin secretion from the pituitary, which in turn activates the ovaries and their sex hormone secretions.

The pulse generator appears to be very sensitive to stress and metabolic factors. In fact, weight loss and severe stress can shut it down completely. It has been well documented that in animals, moderate food restriction or excessive exercise can delay puberty. How the pulse generator knows when to activate is still not known. It is thought that prior to puberty, an inhibition is released by some unknown mechanism, causing the brain to respond to low levels of sex hormones by increasing GnRH stimulation.

Physical and Hormonal Changes

Important changes in body shape and size occur at puberty, all of which may affect the athlete.

One of the first physiologic indications of reproductive maturity is weight gain, particularly in girls who start to secrete estrogen at 9 or 10 years of age. Over the next 2 to 3 years, most girls undergo a relatively dramatic increase in body fat—an average of 11 kg, or about 24 lbs. By the time they reach high school, girls who are not especially athletic will normally have 20% to 27% body fat. This is due to increases in sex hormone secretion, especially estrogen (see Figure 2.1).

Breast and Body Hair Development

Signs of estrogen secretion include breast development and eventually a menstrual period. Male hormones are also secreted at this time, and there is a progressive rise in testosterone and other androgens such as androstenedione and dehydroepiandrosterone sulfate. This is due to adrenarche, or the development of body hair caused by an increase in hormones from the adrenal gland, which occurs before or occasionally at

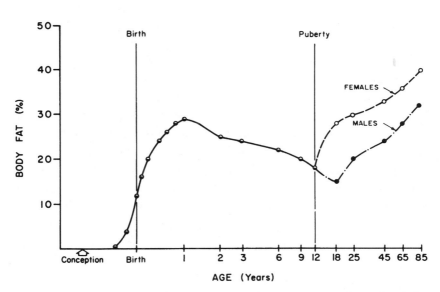

Figure 2.1 *Changing body composition from gestation through adult life. (Reproduced by permission from Bray GA. Major Problems in Internal Medicine, Vol. 9. Philadelphia: W.B. Saunders, 1976.)*

the same time as development of the breasts. The male hormones are responsible for the development of pubic and axillary hair.

Although the initiating components of breast and body hair development are unknown, a large individual variation has been noted among normal girls, suggesting that there may be independent central mechanisms. An unidentified pituitary adrenal-androgen-stimulating hormone may be responsible for adrenarche. Recent study of the hormones that stimulate the adrenal gland, specifically adrenocorticotropin (ACTH), indicates that they are secreted in association with brain peptides that contain opioid-like properties. These include β-endorphin and β-lipotropin, or fragments of these, which may in fact modulate adrenal secretion of androgens, in particular dehydroepiandrosterone (DHEA), one of the first hormones to increase in puberty. These hormones, including β-endorphin, DHEA, and its sulfated derivative (DHEAS), increase with stress. β-endorphin is known to be secreted with ACTH, a pituitary hormone intimately involved with the stress response. This may account for a type of athletically induced delay in puberty and secondary amenorrhea, which is different from the amenorrhea seen with low body weight.

The secretion of estrogen, in particular estradiol from the ovary, determines the onset of thelarche, or breast development. Other factors may also be important, in particular the secretion of hormones such as prolactin from the anterior pituitary gland. Common indices used to determine if estrogen secretion is present include body fat distribution, breast development, bone maturation, vaginal cell cornification, cervical mucous, proliferative endometrium present on biopsy, withdrawal bleeding after the administration of progesterone, and plasma estradiol measurement. The presence of a cornified vaginal smear and bone age are particularly valuable in assessing estrogen secretion in the adolescent girl.

The first few cycles after menarche are usually irregular and anovulatory, but the precise incidence of this phenomenon is not known. This interval of irregularity may last from 1 to 3 years and is generally followed by normal cycles.

The Growth Spurt

A growth spurt also occurs prior to menarche; if it is significantly delayed, obesity may result. Females grow a mean of 25 cm during puberty, with the most rapid growth occurring prior to the first menstrual periods. Growth slows down rapidly after menarche, and the growth potential of postmenarcheal girls is limited. A change in body proportions also occurs at this time. The upper-to-lower (U/L) ratio (defined as length from top of pubic ramus to top of head divided by distance from top of pubic ramus to floor) changes in early puberty because of elongation of the extremities. Later the growth spurt marks a period of equal growth for both torso and lower extremities so that the mean U/L ratio decreases. These changes may be very disconcerting to the young athlete. Growth hormone secretion from the anterior pituitary and gonadal sex hormones appears to be important for regulation of these changes, although the initiating factors are still unknown. Adrenal androgens also may play a role, albeit a less important one.

Bone changes occur during puberty, specifically epiphyseal fusion of different bone centers and osseous maturation, which are evident in x-rays. Bone age is an accurate index of physiologic maturation and correlates closely with pubertal development. It is a valuable tool in the evaluation of children with delayed puberty and can also be used to predict final height.

Bibliography

1. Ferin M, Jewelewicz R, Warren MP. The menstrual cycle. New York: Oxford, 1993.

CHAPTER 3

The Athlete at Puberty and Adolescence

Reproductive Problems (Delayed Puberty)

The effect of exercise and physical training in adolescence has received considerable attention in the medical and sports medicine press. The beneficial effects of exercise are well known, but significant negative effects on the reproductive system can also occur, namely a delay in pubertal development and menarche. The incidence differs widely depending on the athletic discipline but is particularly common in ballet dancers (see Table 3.1).

Primary amenorrhea is defined by a delay in menarche beyond age 16. Many of the variables that are thought to be causal in the menstrual delay—including low body weight or body fat, high levels of physical training, genetic predisposition, dieting behavior, quantity and quality of diet, stress, and amount of training prior to the first period—are present in ballet dancers. There are compelling reasons to suspect that a combination of hereditary and environmental (physical, metabolic, and social) factors may be operative in the phenomenon of delayed menarche. Hereditary influences probably include familial predisposition for delayed menarche, preselection of certain body types for ballet, and low body weight; environmental influences include dieting to maintain low body weight, as well as amount, intensity, and timing of training. Studies have shown that dieting behavior, coupled with associated leanness, leads to an increase in eating disorders, particularly in dancers who have a high incidence of obesity in the family; dieting behavior is also causally related to the delayed menarche and amenorrhea that is so common in this group. Some studies maintain that certain sports favor a specific physique that

13

Table 3.1 *Age of menarche in athletes of different sports*

Sport	Study	n	Average Age (in Years)
Control (in U.S.)	Zacharias et al (1976)	633	12.8
Ballet dancing	Warren and Brooks-Gunn (1989)	64[a]	13.3
	Frisch et al (1980)	69	13.7
	Abraham et al (1982)	29	14.8
Running	Dale et al (1979)	90	12.9
	Frisch et al (1981)	17	13.8
Track and field	Malina et al (1973)	66	13.6
Volleyball	Malina et al (1978)	18	14.2
Skating	Warren and Brooks-Gunn (1989)	25[b]	13.6
Swimming	Fauno et al (1991)	107	12.6
	Warren and Brooks-Gunn (1989)	72[c]	12.9
	Constantini et al (1993)	51[d]	13.8
	Stager and Hatler (1988)	140	14.2

[a] 25% were premenarcheal
[b] 24% were premenarcheal
[c] 4% were premenarcheal
[d] 26% were premenarcheal
Reproduced by permission from Constantini NW, Warren MP. Physical activity, fitness and reproductive health in women. In: Bouchard C, Shephard RJ, Stephens T, eds. Physical activity, fitness and health 1992 proceedings, Champaign, IL: Human Kinetics Publishers, 1994:955–966, p. 956.

in itself predisposes girls to a delay in pubertal development. Others believe that the demands of training represent a delaying force irrespective of physique (they point to the fact that reproductive problems surface particularly at times of heavy training), and still others suggest that the effects may be combined. Another theory maintains that children who have a delay in pubertal development are socialized into competitive athletics.

Recent work has suggested that athletes in some sports that are associated with a prevalence of low body weight have a delay in their first period that differs in mechanism from the delay experienced by athletes in sports in which low body weight is not an issue.

Delay in Puberty and Low Body Weight in Athletes

The ability to remain slender varies considerably from individual to individual and is probably genetically determined. Those athletes or performers who cannot easily keep their weight down are forced to diet strenuously and are vulnerable to reproductive problems, particularly delayed menarche. Problems occur for the female athlete participating in highly competitive activities such as gymnastics, long-distance and cross-country running, skiing, ballet, or figure skating. These girls are often urged to reduce their body fat to less than 10% of their total body weight.

The incidence of delayed menarche varies widely, occurring in 5% to 40% of ballet dancers. Some dancers may not have their first period until as late as their early twenties. Generally, growth is not affected, distinguishing this syndrome from constitutional delay of puberty, but growth may be compromised if an eating disorder is present as well. Each year of training prior to menarche has been related to a delay in menarche of 4 months.

Athletes with delayed menarche usually weigh much less than their peers. One study of dancers showed that the advancement of pubertal stages occurred during times of rest, revealing evidence of a training and activity effect (see Figure 3.1). This effect was all the more impressive because of the rapidity of development during the periods of rest. Normal girls may take an average of 1.9 (± 0.95) years (mean $\pm$ SD) to progress from a Tanner pubertal breast stage 2 to stage 4 (Marshall and Tanner, 1969), whereas in some dancers, an extraordinary progression occurs in as little as 4 months during nonactive intervals. Thus, ballet training during the adolescent years prolongs the prepubertal state and induces primary amenorrhea in dancers (see Figure 3.2). Rest often leads to a striking "catch-up" in puberty. These effects are more notable in women of lower body weight or body fat. However, it is important to note that these individuals who are training heavily and eating marginally do not generally appear malnourished, and there may not be a significant change in weight or body fat during inactive intervals. Rest alone may be sufficient to decrease metabolic demands and promote normal initiation or continuation of sexual development.

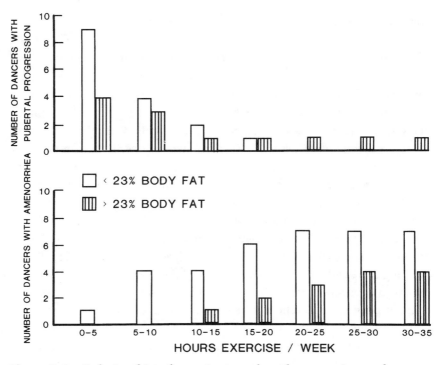

Figure 3.1 *Relationship of exercise to pubertal progression and amenorrhea in ballet dancers. Cumulative data on 15 dancers over a 3-year period of study were gathered on a quarterly basis. The exercise level for the preceding 4 months was averaged on a weekly basis. Differences in weight and body fat were calculated for each quarter preceding and during an event (pubertal progression or amenorrhea). Values did not differ significantly. The top part of the figure includes all dancers including those who developed secondary amenorrhea. Pubertal progression is defined as a change in Tanner stage for breast development or achievement of menarche. (Reproduced by permission from Warren MP. The effects of exercise on pubertal progression and reproductive function in girls. J Clin Endocrinol Metab 1980;51:1150–1157, p. 1153. © The Endocrine Society.)*

The order of pubertal development may also be unusual in ballet dancers. Pubarche, or the development of body hair, is reached at a nearly normal age, but breast development (thelarche) and other estrogen-related factors are suppressed. The large individual variation among normal girls suggests that independent central mechanisms may trigger these two aspects of pubertal development. The fairly normal pubarche and the remarkable delay in thelarche in dancers suggests that the mechanism for pubic hair development either was not affected by—or perhaps was even enhanced by—the large caloric demands, whereas the mechanism affecting both breast development and menarche is definitely suppressed.

Bone age among dancers is delayed, and growth has been noted at as late as 18 and 19 years of age. Long-term effects of a delay in puberty on growth and development are not known. Skeletal measurements of dancers in our study suggest that the delay in menarche may influence long

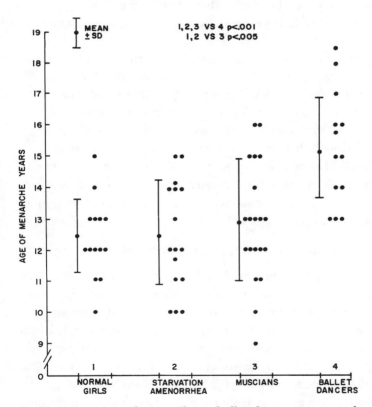

Figure 3.2 *Ages of menarche in ballet dancers compared with those in three other groups. (Reproduced with permission from Warren MP. The effects of exercise on pubertal progression and reproductive function in girls. J Clin Endocrinol Metab 1980;51:1150–1157, p. 1151. © The Endocrine Society.)*

bone growth. The dancers were observed to have a decreased U/L body ratio and a significantly increased arm span compared with the female members of their families. Final heights, however, did not differ. The prolonged hypogonadism (lack of sex hormone secretion) may favor long bone growth, leading to eunuchoidal proportions (long extremities) such as those seen in similar congenital syndromes (for example, sexual immaturity due to lack of pituitary gonadotropic function). Nutritional deprivation may delay epiphyseal closure in the growth centers of the bones (as seen in ballet dancers), although a change in skeletal proportions has not been reported on the basis of nutritional factors alone. The altered skeletal proportions may also be attributable to the fact that ballet attracts girls with these physical characteristics; consequently, they may represent a select group.

Many authors have suggested that the physical characteristics associated with later maturation in females are more suitable for successful athletic performance. One reported group of women with later menarche were more successful runners. Other studies indicate that gymnasts, runners, and other athletes may have characteristic physiques, suggesting a selective phenomenon. It is in fact difficult to know the role inheritance plays in the delay in sexual development. Our studies have suggested that in athletes, particularly dancers, the emphasis on leanness leads to severe dieting; thus the resultant leanness associated with sexual delay is more environmentally than genetically induced.

Delayed Puberty in Athletes with Normal Body Weight

Menstrual dysfunction is common among athletes with very low body mass, such as long-distance runners and dancers, and is usually associated with hypothalamic dysfunction. Recently, another type of menstrual dysfunction has been reported in swimmers, one that is not associated with lower body weight or eating disorders. This appears to be a distinct entity that is less prevalent but is also associated with a delay in menarche. In contrast to the low body weight syndrome, these athletes have normal gonadotropin levels with high luteinizing hormone–follicle-stimulating hormone (LH/FSH) ratios and normal to high estrogen levels. Adrenal hormones, including androstenedione and DHEAS, are higher than in the controls, suggesting increased adrenal stimulation and possible activation of the hypothalamic pituitary adrenal axis. Testosterone levels are also higher. It is unclear whether this mild hyperandrogyneity is exercise-induced or an inherited trait; higher levels of androgens may be self-selecting for this sport or may be stress-induced by activation of the hypothalamic pituitary adrenal axis. The swimmers with a delay in menarche are more prone to irregular cycles later on, but no longitudinal studies exist to indicate whether the hormonal differences persist after exercise is discontinued.

Evaluation

The evaluation of delayed menarche in the setting of exercise should begin with the usual workup for primary amenorrhea: a history of growth and development, breast and pubic hair appearance, weight loss and diet, somatic abnormalities, and exercise training. Some patients will deny weight loss, but continued growth during puberty with a stable weight will constitute a relative weight loss. Physical examination should evaluate weight, height, secondary sexual characteristics, and pelvic or rectal exam. Signs of androgen excess should be noted in particular. Laboratory tests usually include hormonal studies of LH, FSH, prolactin, estradiol levels, and thyroid function; bone age and a CAT scan of the pituitary are done only if indicated. The usual pattern of tests in the athletically induced problem reveals a low estrogen level, normal prolactin, and a low to normal LH and FSH.

A bone age (x-ray of the wrist) is useful to determine potential growth, because a delay in sexual development may be associated with a delay in growth. However, most athletes continue to grow slowly despite a lack of a pubertal growth spurt; severe retardation of growth is unusual. Sophisticated radiographs such as a CAT scan or MRI are indicated if prolactin levels are so elevated as to rule out a pituitary tumor. Gonadal dysgenesis, or Turner's syndrome, which is associated with lack of ovaries, is diagnosed by high LH and FSH levels and a karyotype revealing a 45× chromosome pattern.

Psychological and Physical Aspects

Hyperactivity   All physicians and athletic trainers should be aware of pathologic hyperactivity as a possible sign of anorexia. Certainly young athletes who are training for competition tend to be hyperactive just by virtue of their goals. In the anorectic patient, however, hyperactivity readily becomes uncontrollable, and it may be associated with self-induced vomiting and other forms of purging.

Dieting Behavior   Athletes who need to maintain a low body weight may turn to drastic diets to lower their weight. It has been shown that protein intake may go down, and athletes may consume fewer calories than the RDA (Recommended Daily Allowance). Preoccupation with food (for example, counting peas) is worrisome and may be a precursor of anorexia nervosa. Some athletes may avoid all fat and meat and consume insufficient amounts of iron and other necessary nutrients. Iron-deficient diets are common in vegetarian athletes who do not consume adequate beans and other foods high in iron. Iron deficiency is a particular problem for the growing athlete.

Performance and Effects of Performance-Enhancing Drugs

Anabolic Steroids

Some athletes have turned to anabolic steroids to enhance the size and strength of their muscular system or for motivational effects. These drugs are not legal or approved for such indications, and their use is particularly damaging to young athletes who have not yet completed sexual development or growth. Anabolic steroids may also have dramatic effects on mood, particularly on the unstable personality of the adolescent.

In adolescent women, the most worrisome effects of anabolic steroid use include fusion of the epiphyses (growth plates) and compromise of full height potential. Accelerated sexual development may occur, as well as masculinizing effects such as acne, hirsutism, irregular or absent periods, deepening of the voice, male pattern baldness, and hypertrophy of the clitoris. Aggressive behavior and moodiness are other potential problems, and psychotic behavior has also been reported. Although many of the problems are reversible, voice changes and clitoromegaly are usually permanent. The issues concerning performance-enhancing drugs are covered in detail in Chapter 10.

Growth Hormone

Growth hormone (GH) is known to cause nitrogen retention and a general anabolic effect, the net result of which is an increase in strength, particularly of the muscles. GH is expensive and available only for treating children with short stature due to GH deficiency. It is not approved for use in muscle development but is nonetheless commonly found in the athletic population for this reason. Some athletes believe it will increase height, although its use in the normal non-GH-deficient population has not substantiated this claim. GH can cause carbohydrate intolerance and diabetes. Prepubertal patients with excess GH secretion are known to develop gigantism, weak muscles, osteoporosis, and cardiac failure. The effect of short-term exogenous GH use is unknown.

Medical and Gynecologic Complications

Delayed Maturation with Low Body Weight

Young athletes in this group appear to have fairly specific problems that relate to their low body weight. Female adolescents may develop a behavior pattern that appears to have its roots in early puberty: dieting or restricted eating patterns that in severe cases may lead to physical and psychological problems, including secondary amenorrhea and anorexia nervosa. Special groups, including gymnasts, figure skaters, runners, and in particular ballet dancers, adhere to restrictive eating patterns to achieve the ideal body physique needed to attain maximal performance. Girls participating in these activities have a much higher incidence of anorexia nervosa than is found in the normal population. Puberty is associated with a rapid accumulation of fat, and in view of the important effects of nutrition on menarche, it is extremely likely that nutritional factors play an important role in the marked delay of menarche seen in women pursuing these disciplines. Altered diets have also been reported in runners who began training prior to menarche, and this group also has a higher incidence of anorexia nervosa. Anorexia nervosa, particularly those cases in which body weight falls below 85% of normal, may be accompanied by severe psychological changes, increased morbidity, and a mortality rate of 10%. Morbidity associated with anorexia nervosa includes osteoporosis, fractures, and anemia, as well as a variety of physical signs and symptoms including abdominal pain, intolerance to cold, easy bruisability, bradycardia, hypotension, and severe constipation. Bulimia may also develop in a misguided attempt to keep weight down and may lead to dehydration, cramps, and seizures.

The prolonged hypogonadism seen in athletes may also favor long bone growth, leading to eunuchoidal proportions similar to those seen in hypogonadotropic hypogonadism. Nutritional deprivation may delay epiphyseal closure, as seen in ballet dancers. The effect of prolonged estrogen deficiency on the adolescent is not known. However, recent studies show that hypoestrogenism in young athletic women decreases bone density and increases the possibility of premature osteoporosis and delayed bone maturation. This problem may be compounded by the poor diets these women follow. The adolescent athlete's diet, in addition to being too low in calories, may also be inadequate in fat and fat-soluble vitamins and minerals, particularly vitamin D, calcium, and iron, and may be too high in fiber. This is particularly worrisome in the growing athlete, and supplements may be necessary.

The osteopenia reported in young athletes may be due to lack of bone accretion at puberty rather than bone loss. Recent evidence suggests that bone mass does not reach a normal peak if puberty is very delayed. These young athletes are susceptible to stress fractures as well as scoliosis, which has been reported in 23% of young ballet dancers. Bone that is stressed by use and athletic activity usually increases in density, but this response appears to be absent in the young individual with delayed puberty. Growth at adolescence may produce a fragile skeleton that is inadequately mineralized without sex hormone secretion. Hypoestrogenism may also delay maturation of osseous centers in the spine, leading to a predisposition to vertebral instability and curvature. Collapse of the femoral head (resembling osteonecrosis) was noted in a 20-year-old dancer who had extreme skeletal development delay. Exercise appears to increase bone density only in the presence of normal estrogen secretion, contrary to data reported in postmenopausal women. This may account for the high incidence of stress fractures in young exercising amenorrheic athletes and confirms that a relative osteopenia may exist in this group. An increase in bone has been noted with puberty with this group, but levels still remain significantly below normal.

Treatment

The delay in menarche can usually be reversed by decreasing exercise, increasing weight slightly, or both. Recurrent stress fractures may be a hallmark of dieting behavior; an attempt should be made to identify and treat this problem immediately.

Cyclic estrogen in combination with a progestin should be given in order to prevent bone demineralization if growth is complete. If the epiphyses are not fused, estrogen treatment may close the growth plate and stop further growth. Unfortunately, hormone replacement therapy has not been shown to improve bone mass. However, most physicians would choose to treat until further data are available. Conjugated estrogens (Premarin or its equivalent) are given in doses of 0.625 mg for 25 days with 10 mg of medroxyprogesterone (Provera) added on days 16 to 25. A week without therapy follows. This dosage is thought to prevent further loss of bone mass in athletes with recent amenorrhea but not to replace bone loss that has already occurred following amenorrhea of longer duration. If periods are desired, the patient may need to take 1.25–2.5 mg of Premarin each day. An oral contraceptive in low dose may also be used.

If the athlete is making estrogen withdrawal with Provera, 10 mg for 5 to 10 days every 6 to 8 weeks will be sufficient to prevent overstimulation of the endometrium and prolonged irregular bleeding.

Side effects are unlikely to occur with these very small doses of estrogen, but they might include headaches, elevated blood pressure, and breakthrough bleeding. The long-term consequences of low doses of estrogens (given with progesterone) are as yet unknown.

Bibliography

1. Abraham SF, Beumont PJV, Fraser IS, et al. Body weight, exercise and menstrual status among ballet dancers in training. Br J Obstet Gynaecol 1982;89:507–510.
2. Apter D, Viinikka L, Vikko R. Hormonal pattern of adolescent menstrual cycles. J Clin Endocrinol Metab 1978;47:944–954.
3. Brooks-Gunn J, Attie I, Burrow C, et al. The impact of puberty on body and eating concerns in athletic and nonathletic contexts. J Early Adolesc 1989;9:269–290.
4. Brooks-Gunn J, Warren MP. Mother-daughter differences in menarcheal age in adolescent girls attending national dance company schools and non-dancers. Ann Hum Biol 1988;15:35–43.
5. Brooks-Gunn J, Warren MP, Hamilton LH. The relation of eating problems and amenorrhea in ballet dancers. Med Sci Sports Exerc 1987;19:41–44.
6. Comerci GD. Normal pubescent growth and sexual maturation. Semin Adolesc Med 1987;3:217–226.

7. Constantini WN, Persitz E, Warren MP. Athletic amenorrhea in swimmers: a different mechanism. Med Sci Sports Exerc 1993;25(5):5141.

8. Cutler GBJ, Cassorla FG, Ross JL, et al. Pubertal growth: physiology and pathophysiology. Recent Prog Horm Res 1986;42:443–470.

9. Dale E, Gerlach DH, Wilhite AL. Menstrual dysfunction in distance runners. Obstet Gynecol 1979;54:47–53.

10. Fauno P, Kalund S, Kanstrup IL. Menstrual patterns in Danish elite swimmers. Eur J Appl Physiol 1991;62:36–39.

11. Frisch RE, Gotz-Welbergen AV, McArthur JW. Delayed menarche and amenorrhea of college athletes in relation to age of onset of training. JAMA 1981;246(14):1559–1563.

12. Frisch RE, Wyshak G, Vincent L. Delayed menarche and amenorrhea in ballet dancers. N Engl J Med 1980;303:17–19.

13. Grumbach MM, Roth JC, Kaplan SL, Kelch RP. Hypothalamic pituitary regulation of puberty in man: evidence and concepts derived from clinical research. In: Grumbach MM, Grave D, Mayer FF, eds. Control of the onset of puberty. New York: Wiley, 1974:115–166.

14. Malina RM, Harper AB, Avent HH, et al. Age at menarche in athletes and non-athletes. Med Sci Sports Exerc 1973;5(1):11–13.

15. Malina RM, Spirduso WW, Tate C, et al. Age at menarche and selected menstrual characteristics in athletes at different competitive levels and in different sports. Med Sci Sports Exerc 1978;10(3):218–222.

16. Marshall WA, Tanner JM. Variations in pattern of pubertal changes in girls. Arch Dis Childh 1969;44:291–303.

17. Odell WD. The physiology of puberty: disorders of the pubertal process. In: DeGroot LJ, ed. Endocrinology. New York: Grune and Stratton, 1979:1163–1379.

18. Reiter EO, Kulin HE. Sexual maturation in the female—normal development and precocious puberty. Pediatr Clin North Am 1972;19:581–603.

19. Stager JM, Hatler LK. Menarche in athletes: the influence of genetics and prepubertal training. Med Sci Sports Exerc 1988;20(4):369–373.

20. Styne DM, Grumbach MM. Puberty in the male and the female; its physiology and disorders. In: Yen SSC, Jaffe RB, eds. Reproductive endocrinology: physiology, pathophysiology and clinical management. Philadelphia: WB Saunders, 1978:234–235.

21. Warren MP. The effects of exercise on pubertal progression and reproductive function in girls. J Clin Endocrinol Metab 1980;51:1150–1157.

22. Warren MP. Excessive dieting and exercise: the dangers for young athletes. J Musculoskel Med 1987;4:31–40.

23. Warren MP. Anorexia nervosa and eating disorders. In: Kelley WN, ed. Textbook of internal medicine. Philadelphia: JB Lippincott, 1989:2284–2286.

24. Warren MP. Metabolic factors and the onset of puberty. In: Grumbach MM, Sizonenko PC, Aubert MA, eds. The control of the onset of puberty II. Baltimore: Williams & Wilkins, 1989:553–575.

25. Warren MP. Reproductive function in the ballet dancer. In: Pirke KM, Wuttke W, Schweiger U, eds. The menstrual cycle and its disorders: influences of nutrition, exercise and neurotransmitters. Berlin: Springer-Verlag, 1989:161–170.

26. Warren MP, Brooks-Gunn J. Delayed menarche in athletes: the role of low energy intake and eating disorders and their relation to bone density. In: Laron Z, Rogol AD, eds. Hormones and sport; vol. 55. New York: Serono Symposia Publications, 1989:41–54.

27. Warren MP, Brooks-Gunn J, Hamilton LH, et al. Scoliosis and fractures in young ballet dancers: relation to delayed menarche and secondary amenorrhea. N Engl J Med 1986;314:1348–1353.

28. Zacharias L, Rand WM, Wurtman RJ. A prospective study of sexual development and growth in American girls: the statistics of menarche. Obstet Gynecol Surv 1976;31:325–337.

CHAPTER 4

The Female Reproductive System and the Normal Menstrual Cycle

T he effects of exercise on the normal cycling woman are more easily understood once the normal reproductive tract and the physiology of the menstrual cycle are reviewed. Multiple hormonal events that are easily affected by physical stress will be addressed in subsequent chapters.

The Reproductive Axis

The entire reproductive system in the woman includes the hypothalamic area and the pituitary in the brain as well as the ovaries and associated organs (see Figure 4.1). The two ovaries, which are filled with follicles, are adjacent to the two fallopian tubes, which emanate from the uterus. The lower end of the uterus, the cervix, leads to the vagina. The endometrium, or lining, of the uterus undergoes extensive changes during the menstrual cycle and is shed during menstruation.

The target organ for the hypothalamic pituitary axis system is, of course, the ovaries. Overstimulation of the target organ is prevented by a feedback system, in which the response of the end organ (ovary) shuts down the signals from the hypothalamus and pituitary. This is called negative feedback. In addition, the end organ may elicit a stimulatory or positive response from the hypothalamus in order to signal that hormone levels are ready for ovulation. These signals are very sensitive to environmental stresses such as weight loss or exercise. The hypothalamus exerts a signal to the pituitary by means of the secretion of GnRH and the pituitary by means of secretion of LH and FSH. The principal secretions of the ovary are estrogens, particularly estradiol; progestins, especially

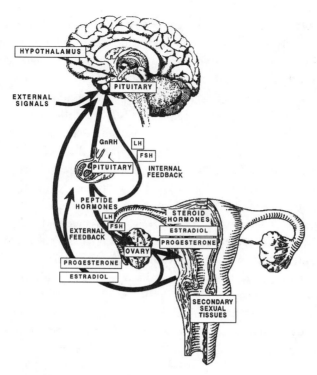

Figure 4.1 *View of the entire female reproductive system. Reprinted with permission from Diagnostic Products Corporation.*

progesterone; and androgens. Estradiol and progesterone appear to be the main ovarian steroids of the menstrual cycle (Figure 4.2).

The Menstrual Cycle

The menstrual cycle is divided into two phases: the follicular, or preovulatory phase, and the luteal, or postovulatory phase. An orderly sequence of events during the maturation of the follicle is associated with changes in the women's reproductive tract. This sequence can occur only when very specific pulses of GnRH, occurring every 60 to 90 minutes, stimulate the pituitary, which in turn releases bursts of LH and FSH.

A new cycle begins when the uterus sheds the endometrium (menses). By convention, day 1 of the cycle is considered the first day of visible bleeding. On day 1 the size of the largest follicle is 3 to 4 mm; a few days later a dominant follicle starts to emerge and clearly grows faster than the others. The development of this dominant follicle is first signaled by a fall in estrogen levels, which occurs with the end of the previous cycle. This fall initiates a negative feedback effect on the hypothalamic pituitary axis, causing a rise in FSH levels. Granulosa cells in the follicle then increase in number by mitotic division, thereby increasing the number of FSH receptors; these in turn acquire aromatase activity and develop the ability to synthesize estradiol. The rising estradiol levels eventually suppress FSH levels. LH receptors also appear in the granulosa cells as a result of combined FSH and estradiol activity; they increase estradiol levels by stimulating aromatizable androgens to estrogens in the thecal area of the follicle. A surge of estradiol occurs, which causes release of LH and FSH from the pituitary (positive feedback), which causes ovulation. The mature follicle is released and makes its way into the fallopian tube.

Ovulation marks the end of the follicular phase and the beginning of the luteal phase. The empty follicle in the ovary starts to vascularize, and luteal cells develop and start to make estrogen and progesterone, forming the corpus luteum. The corpus luteum usually has a finite span of 14 days. With the fall in estrogen and progesterone levels, the corpus luteum involutes, and a new cycle begins (Figure 4.2). Progesterone is the dominant hormone in the luteal phase and causes a secretory change in the endometrial glands. Each event is intricately involved with the next, and the entire process may be altered by changes in one of the signals or the response of the ovary. The key signals to the ovary from the hypothalamic pituitary axis are the stimulating effects of LH and FSH. Both these hormones are necessary for follicle development and ovulation.

The way in which these hormones are secreted is also very important. As mentioned, both gonadotropins are secreted from the pituitary in very precise pulses as a result of similar signals from the hypothalamus. This organ secretes GnRH, which is programmed to be delivered in bursts every 60 to 90 minutes. The numbers of pulses, as well as their amplitude, may change during the menstrual cycle, but the pulsatility remains key to the development of the normal follicle. The mechanisms that initiate and maintain these pulses are poorly understood but are definitely affected by higher centers which are influenced by external stimuli, including stress and exercise. The so-called pulse generator is located in an area of the

FSH Follicular Stimulating Hormone

FSH is produced by the beta cells of the anterior pituitary gland. FSH is important in the development and maintenance of gonadal tissues that secrete steroid hormones and is controlled by negative feedback from these steroids. FSH initiates growth and development of the ovarian follicles. In menopause, FSH increases due to diminished ovarian function associated with decreased Estradiol levels.

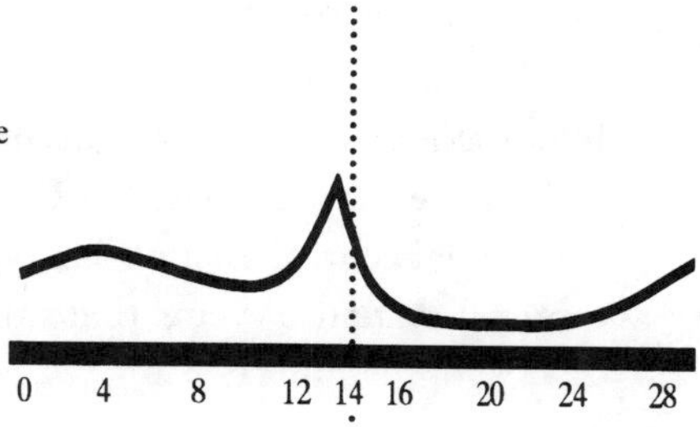

LH Luteinizing Hormone

LH is also produced by the pituitary gland, and promotes ovulation in the mature follicle and steroid production by the corpus luteum. Ovulation occurs within a 48-hour window bracketing the LH peak during the midcycle surge. LH increases in menopause in response to decreasing Estradiol and Progesterone levels. This increasing LH trend is reversed with estrogen replacement therapy. LH and growth hormone are the first hormones affected by pituitary diseases.

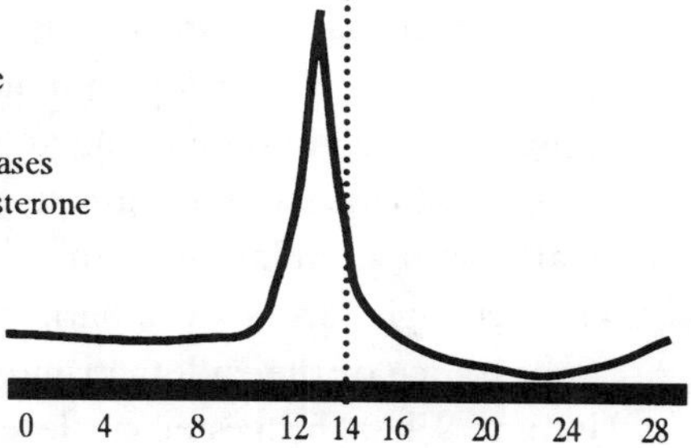

Estradiol

ESTRADIOL is the most potent estrogen and is produced by the ovaries. Estradiol measurements are used principally for monitoring ovulation induction and in the differential diagnosis of amenorrhea. Estradiol has also proven to be of value in evaluating precocious puberty in girls. During the menstrual cycle, preovulatory levels rise to indicate the degree of follicular maturation, and decrease at the end of the luteal phase prior to the onset of menses.

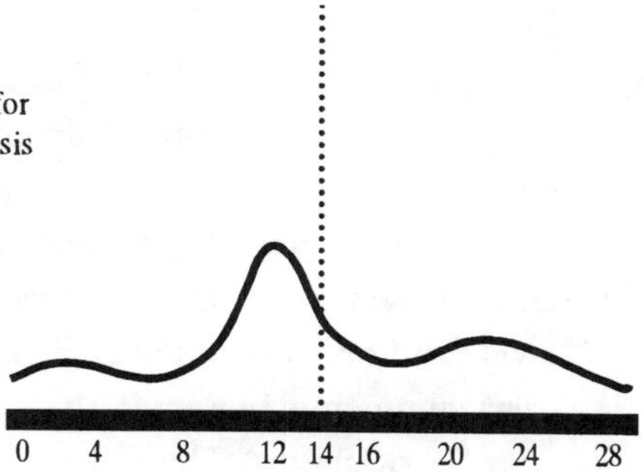

Progesterone

PROGESTERONE is a steroid hormone which plays an important role in the preparation for and maintenance of pregnancy. It is produced in the ovaries (corpus luteum), placenta and small amounts in the adrenal cortex. Along with Estradiol, Progesterone helps control the phases of the menstrual cycle. Progesterone remains at a baseline level throughout the follicular phase and begins to rise during the LH surge. This stimulates the uterine lining in readiness for embryo implantation and Progesterone levels continue to rise during normal pregnancy. If pregnancy does not occur the Progesterone level drops off, and the cycle starts over.

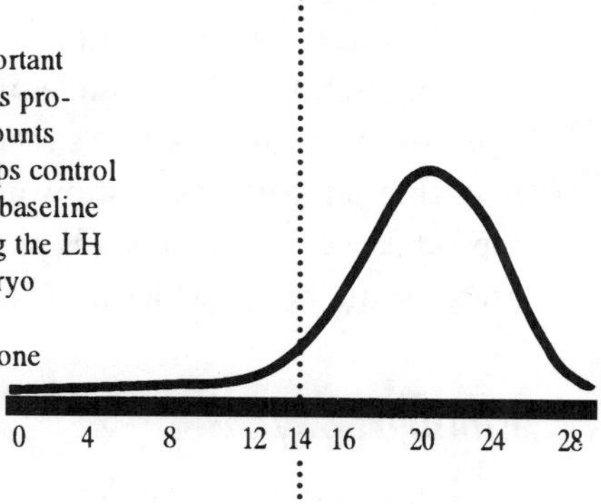

Figure 4.2 *Changes in hormone levels during the menstrual cycle. Reprinted with permission from Diagnostic Products Corporation.*

hypothalamus called the arcuate nucleus, where neurons containing GnRH are situated. The GnRH travels down the axon of the neurons to the medial central area of the hypothalamus; from there it is released into a portal system of veins that takes it to the pituitary (see Figure 4.1).

The Reproductive Tract

During the menstrual cycle, important changes occur in the reproductive tract, particularly in the uterus. During the follicular phase, the endometrial lining grows rapidly with multiple mitotic divisions. The thickness of the endometrium is determined by the length of estrogen stimulation. The growth of the endometrium stops with ovulation, and a secretory phase starts with stimulation of the glands and the accumulation of glycogen. The changes are so dramatic that one can tell from the microscopic appearance of the endometrium how many days have elapsed since ovulation. When progesterone levels fall because of failure of the corpus luteum, collapse of the vascular supply causes the endometrium to shed along a fairly precise line of cleavage. If pregnancy occurs, human chorionic gonadotropin (hCG) from the embryo will sustain progesterone secretion from the corpus luteum.

The cervix may also experience changes, including the development of clear watery mucous at midcycle due to the influence of high estrogen levels and opening of the os. The glycoprotein filaments that make up the cervical mucous line up fairly precisely at this time, probably to allow the passage of sperm. The fallopian tubes, which contain ciliae, have been noted to start beating more frequently immediately after ovulation, presumably to allow the passage of the fertilized ovum into the uterus. The walls of the vagina contain superficial cells that change in appearance and may clump together and show accumulation of glycogen. Thus, the entire reproductive system depends on the interaction of hormones from diverse areas of the body, which change daily and even from minute to minute.

Bibliography

1.   Ferin M, Jewelewicz R, Warren MP. The menstrual cycle. New York: Oxford, 1993.

The Adult Athlete: Reproductive Problems

Amenorrhea and Irregular Periods

The athlete has a higher than normal incidence of irregular periods and amenorrhea (no periods for more than 6 months). These problems appear to have multiple genetic and environmental causes (nutrition, weight loss, stress) and occur more frequently in younger athletes whose reproductive systems are not fully mature. Sometimes the abnormalities are very minor and are due to a lengthening of the preovulatory (follicular) phase or a shortening of the postovulatory (luteal) phase. Thus, athletes may experience longer intervals between periods, shorter intervals, or no periods at all.

The prevalence of menstrual problems varies but has been reported to be 2% to 20% in runners (50% in elite runners) and 30% to 50% in professional dancers. One study of marathon runners showed a 7% incidence of amenorrhea, mostly in women who weighed less and were slightly younger. Several studies have shown a correlation between training intensity and reproductive dysfunction, although other studies did not. Amenorrhea in runners does not appear to increase simply upon increasing mileage, although this problem is much more frequent in highly competitive environments.

This problem appears to be due to a hypothalamic dysfunction or a decrease in the pulses of GnRH from the hypothalamus (see Figure 5.1), which in turn lowers LH and FSH secretion and shuts down stimulation to the ovary. Occasionally a reversion to pubertal and prepubertal types of LH secretion occurs with spiking of LH pulses at night. Initially, at the start of training, one can see inadequate luteal phases with a shortened

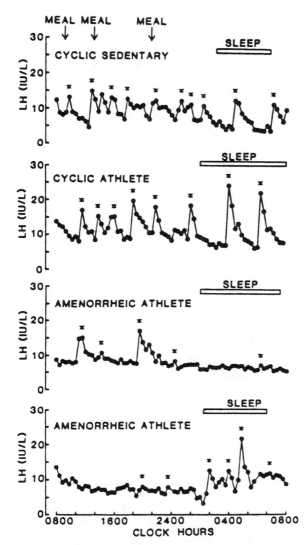

Figure 5.1 *Athletic training and the menstrual cycle. Exercise influences pulsatile LH activity in women athletes; the severity of the inhibition depends on the strenuousness of the exercise and the particular sensitivity of each individual. With ongoing function of the GnRH pulse generator, the athlete continues to have normal ovulatory menstrual cycles. Menstrual cycle disturbances parallel the severity of the decrease in pulse frequency. (Reproduced by permission from Loucks AB, Mortola JF, Girton L, Yen SSC. Alterations in the hypothalamic-pituitary-ovarian and the hypothalamic-pituitary-adrenal axes in athletic women. J Clin Endocrinol Metab 1989;68:402–411, p. 407. © The Endocrine Society.)*

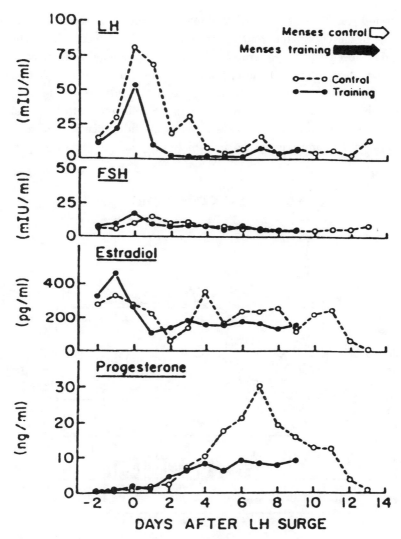

Figure 5.2 *Short luteal phase in a long-distance runner. Abnormal progesterone secretion (short or inadequate luteal phase) may follow deficiencies in gonadotropin secretion and in follicular maturation. In this example, the cycle during training (solid circles) is characterized by a short luteal phase. (Reproduced by permission from Shangold M, Freeman R, Thysen B, Gatz M. The relationship between long-distance running plasma progesterone and luteal phase length. Fertil Steril 1979;31:130–133, p. 131.)*

cycle (see Figure 5.2) or just a lack of ovulation, but some athletes may shut down completely and progress to complete amenorrhea. The problem has been difficult to reproduce in normal women; normal women who were given intensive training showed only minor problems that were more frequent if some weight loss also occurred (see Figure 5.3). In fact, this type of hypothalamic dysfunction is more frequent in athletes with low body weight, as are found in endurance sports, such as marathon running, or sports in which low weight enhances per-

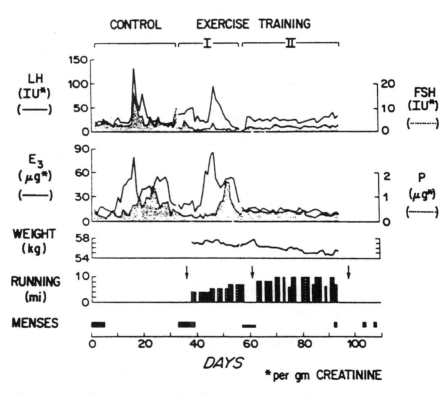

Figure 5.3   *Three sequential cycles in a woman who began as sedentary (control cycle) and was running nearly 10 miles per day by cycle 2. Urinary hormone concentrations show probable luteal phase shortening in cycle 1 and loss of estradiol and LH surges in cycle 2. (Reproduced by permission from Bullen BA, Skrinar GS, Beitins IZ, et al. Induction of menstrual disorders by strenuous exercise in untrained women. N Engl J Med 1985;312:1349–1353, p. 1352.)*

formance or aesthetic appeal, such as ballet dancing, gymnastics, and figure skating.

A popular theory has maintained that low body fat is the cause of amenorrhea, and 22% body fat is thought to be necessary for maintenance of regular cycles. This variable has been increasingly challenged as a causal mechanism, however. Regular cycles are seen in athletes with less than 17% body fat, and amenorrheic and eumenorrheic runners have been found to have similar percentages of body fat. Thus, the fact that reproductive dysfunction is not commonly seen in athletes who have a high percentage of body fat probably reflects metabolic parameters other than weight or percentage of body fat. Weight loss, however, can profoundly affect cycles in athletes (see Table 5.1).

Other associated factors seen with endurance training include the intensity of training, diet (or energy and nutrition), decreased basal metabolic rate, and training before menarche. The most popular theories for the mechanism of all athletic amenorrhea suggest that an energy drain may exist during training, when caloric intake decreases and energy output

Table 5.1 *Incidence of luteal phase defects and anovulation* in the general population,[†] and in 28 young women who participated in a prospective progressive increase in vigorous exercise with or without weight loss*

Abnormal Cycle	General Population[‡]	Vigorous Exercise[§] During a 4-Week Span	
		No Weight Loss	Weight Loss
Luteal phase defects	15.8%	33%	63%
Anovulation	10.6%	42%	81%

* Loss of luteinizing hormone surge or flat basal body temperature.
[†] Ages 20 to 30, 1004 cycles.
[‡] Weighted mean from Collet ME, et al. Fertil Steril 1954;5:437; Doring GK, J Reprod Fertil Suppl 1969;6:77; and Metcalf MG, et al. J Endocrinol 1983;97:213.
[§] Data from Bullen BA, Skrinar GS, Beitins IZ, et al. Induction of menstrual disorders in untrained women by strenuous exercise. N Engl J Med 1985;312:1349.
Reproduced by permission from Yen SSC. Chronic anovulation due to CNS-hypothalamic-pituitary dysfunction. In: Yen SSC, Jaffe RB, eds. Reproductive endocrinology, 3rd ed. Philadelphia: WB Saunders, 1991:631–688, p. 667.

cannot be met. Recent physiologic experiments on normal women suggest that reproductive hormones (measured by LH pulsatility) are not affected in exercising women until nutrition is restricted. Thus, a physiologic paradox exists: a large energy output is not compensated for by increased caloric intake yet weight loss does not occur. Thus, training appears to be associated with increased caloric efficiency and may represent an adaptive syndrome. Initial studies examining energy balance are conflicting. A number of studies have found that resting metabolic rate increases during an exercise training program (with an increase in dietary intake); others have shown no effect of training on resting metabolic rate. Still others have speculated that restrictions in diet and intense exercise deplete energy stores, stimulating the body to increase food efficiency by decreasing metabolic rate. How these adaptive changes tie in with reproductive dysfunction is unclear, but the well-documented decreases in GnRH pulses suggest that the GnRH pulse generator may be affected by metabolic fuels. Another theory suggests that activation of the hypothalamic pituitary adrenal axis suppresses the GnRH pulse generator. The hypothalamic hormone CRF (corticotropin releasing factor), which stimulates ACTH, has been shown to suppress GnRH pulses. ACTH and cortisol levels are elevated during exercise, and disturbances of both ACTH and cortisol rhythms have been found in amenorrheic runners. This may be a side effect of the activation of CRF, which may be the factor that suppresses GnRH. Thus, it has been hypothesized that the stress of chronic exercise or competition may be the initiating factor that induces reproductive dysfunction. Alternatively, this type of amenorrhea may be different from that seen with an energy drain or may be superimposed on it.

The type of menstrual dysfunction that is seen in endurance sports and in sports in which low body weight is an advantage should be differentiated from the menstrual dysfunction seen in other sports, such as swimming. The incidence of complete amenorrhea is lower in sports not associated with low body weight (see Figure 5.4), and menses are more often irregular. Menstrual irregularity can occur with increased LH levels, increased LH/FSH ratios, normal estrogen levels, and higher levels of androgens, in particular DHEAS (see Table 5.2). This problem has been reported in swimmers and may represent an anovulatory syndrome that resembles, in terms of the hormonal profile, the polycystic ovarian

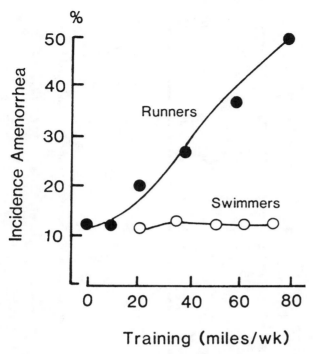

Figure 5.4 *Among runners, the frequency of amenorrhea was positively correlated with the number of miles run per week. In contrast, among swimmers, in endurance training the frequency of amenorrhea was about 12% and was independent of the intensity of training. (Reproduced by permission from Sanborn CF, Martin BJ, Wagner WW Jr. Is athletic amenorrhea specific to runners? Am J Obstet Gynecol 1982;143:859–861, p. 860.)*

syndrome. Stress, which may elevate androgens, may be the causal mechanism, but more work is needed to further define this problem.

Recent literature has begun to examine the frequency with which eating disorders occur in the athletic population. Eating disorders have recently been recognized as a contributing cause of the so-called athletic amenorrhea and are part of the clinical symptom complex known as "the female athletic triad," which consists of amenorrhea, eating disorders, and osteoporosis. Eating disorders may occur initially as chronic dieting to try to lower weight but may progress to full-blown anorexia or bulimia.

Table 5.2 *Hormone concentration in swimmers according to menstrual status*

Menstrual Group (n)	LH (mIU)	FSH (mIU)	LH/FSH (ratio)	E2 (pg/ml)	Test (ng/dl)	A (ng/dl)	DHEAS (ng/dl)
Premenarche Athletes (9)	15.3 ± 1.7[a]	10.6 ± 0.9[a]	1.5 ± 0.2	14.4 ± 12[a]	53.3 ± 4.1[b]	179 ± 18	170.3 ± 23[a]
Nonathletes (80)	1.6 ± 0.1	2.8 ± 0.1	—	34.4 ± 4.0	41.4 ± 2.1	—	100.2 ± 6.0
Postmenarche Athletes: Regular (6)	20.5 ± 2.9[a]	10.1 ± 1.2[a]	1.9 ± 0.4	67.2 ± 10	60.0 ± 6.8	200 ± 23	388.0 ± 59[b]
Athletes: Irregular[c] (9)	16.7 ± 1.7[a]	11.2 ± 1.3[a]	1.6 ± 0.2	80.6 ± 7	63.3 ± 6.5	205 ± 16	257.7 ± 34[b]
Nonathletes (41)	2.8 ± 0.3	4.5 ± 0.3	—	85.2 ± 10.5	61.3 ± 4.6	121 (80–300)[d]	174.3 ± 12.2

Data summarized as mean ± SE (range in parentheses).
Normal levels for all hormones except A are taken from Warren and Brooks-Gunn 1989.
Statistical significance are for swimmers compared with nonathletes.
[a] $p < 0.0001$
[b] $p < 0.05$
[c] Irregular = oligomenorrhea and amenorrhea
[d] Normal levels of A are taken from Winter et al 1978.
Reproduced by permission from Constantini NW, Warren MP. Menstrual dysfunction in swimmers: a distinct entity. J Clin Endocrinol Metab 1995;80:2740–2744, p. 2742. © The Endocrine Society.

Workup of the Menstrual Dysfunction Seen in Athletes

Short Cycles, Long Cycles, or Irregular Bleeding   These women generally have a longer follicular phase or absence of a critical hormone surge (estradiol, LH) at midcycle that prevents or delays ovulation. Alternatively, ovulation may have occurred, but due to inadequate follicular development there is poor corpus luteum function, resulting in a short luteal phase and low progesterone levels. Women typically report that they have recently increased their exercise, and the problem is easily reversed with a decrease in training. A physical and pelvic examination should include examination for virilization including hirsutism, acne, clitoromegaly, and galactorrhea. Hormone evaluation is generally limited to a pregnancy test or, if the problem is of long duration (6 months), a prolactin and LH/FSH level. A blood BHCG test commonly done in pregnancy measures one of the subunits of the hormone human chorionic gonadotropin secreted in pregnancy. Although DHEAS may be elevated in women with an anovulatory syndrome, it is not out of the range of normal. Thus, watchful waiting is permissible if the training season is about to end. Excessive or lack of bleeding may be a problem and can be treated with a progestin such as Provera for 5 to 10 days. Alternatively, oral contraceptives can be used to return the athlete's cycle to normal.

Complete Amenorrhea   Physical and pelvic examination is again indicated to rule out androgenization, galactorrhea, and pregnancy. A careful history of weight loss and eating disorders should be taken. It is worth noting that athletes who are vegetarians have a higher incidence of problems. Complete amenorrhea surfaces in exercising women if their weight is less than 90% of ideal. A hormonal evaluation should include an LH/FSH level and a BHCG pregnancy test. Often the estradiol level is tested to determine the extent of the hypothalamic suppression. Typically, in the amenorrhea associated with endurance exercise and as low weight LH is selectively more suppressed than FSH, and the estradiol level is low. A prolactin level will rule out a pituitary adenoma, and FSH and LH levels will rule out ovarian failure. In rare cases, hyper- or hypothyroidism may be associated with amenorrhea, so thyroid function tests are generally done. The diagnosis of an eating disorder will generally be missed unless specifically searched for, because of the strong pattern of denial.

A standardized scale or a diagnostic interview must be obtained if the diagnosis is unclear.

Eating Disorders   Anorexia nervosa may be diagnosed in the athlete when weight loss is severe. In this syndrome, a classic triad occurs with amenorrhea, weight loss, and a psychiatric disturbance. It is now well recognized that some athletic disciplines present risk factors for the development of eating disorders and amenorrhea, particularly when low

Table 5.3 *Prevalence of eating disorders in different athletic disciplines*

Activity	Study	n	Percentage with Eating Disorder
Nonathletes	Borgen and Corbin (1987)	101	6
Activities emphasizing leanness			
Dancing	Brooks-Gunn et al (1987)	55	33
Combined activities	Borgen and Corbin (1987)	33	20
Gymnastics	Rosen et al (1986)	19	74
Track	Rosen et al (1986)	40	35
Activities not emphasizing leanness			
Combined activities	Borgen and Corbin (1987)	32	0
Tennis	Rosen et al (1986)	25	24
Volleyball	Rosen et al (1986)	14	21

Reproduced by permission from Constantini NW, Warren MP. Special problems of the female athlete. In: Panush RS, ed. Exercise and rheumatic disease, Bailliere's Clinical Rheumatology Series, London: Bailliere Tindall, 1994:199–219, p. 213.
Borgen JS, Corbin CB. Eating disorders among female athletes. The Physician and Sportsmedicine 1987;15(2):89–95.
Brooks-Gunn J, Warren MP, Hamilton LH. The relationship of eating disorders to amenorrhoea in ballet dancers. Medicine and Science in Sports and Exercise 1987;19(1):41–44.
Rosen LW, McKeag DB, Hough DO, Curley V. Pathogenic weight-control behavior in female athletes. The Physician and Sportsmedicine 1986;14(1):79–86.

Table 5.4   *Symptoms and signs of anorexia nervosa*

	Total No.	Percentage	Reported in Starvation*
Amenorrhea (22 postpubertal girls)	22/22	101.0	Yes
Constipation	26/42	61.9	Yes
Preoccupation with food	19/42	45.2	Yes
Abdominal pain	8/42	19.0	Yes
Intolerance to cold	8/42	19.0	Yes
Vomiting	5/42	4.9	No
Hypotension	36/42	85.7	Yes
Hypothermia	27/42	64.3	Yes
Dry skin	26/42	61.9	Yes
Lanugo-type hair	22/42	52.4	Yes
Bradycardia	11/42	26.2	Yes
Edema	11/42	26.2	Yes
Systolic murmur	6/42	14.3	No
Petechiae	4/42	9.5	Yes

* The symptoms enumerated are also seen during periods of starvation.
Reproduced by permission from Warren MP. Eating, body weight and menstrual function. In: Brownell KD, Rodin J, Wilmore JH, eds. Eating, body weight and performance in athletes: disorders of modern society, Philadelphia: Lea & Febiger, 1992:222–234, p. 229.

weight is emphasized (see Table 5.3). The incidence of anorexia nervosa in ballet dancers ranges from 1 in 5 to 1 in 20 (see Figure 5.5). Weight loss is usually 25% below ideal. The psychiatric disturbance includes a disturbance of perception with a distorted view of the body, generally with an unreasonable concern about being "too fat." These women are often hyperactive and might engage in strenuous sports such as long-distance running. They may count peas and grams of cereal and overuse artificial sweetners. Diverse physical changes occur, which are generally thought to be due to a physical and metabolic adaptation to the semistarved state. Common signs are listed in Table 5.4. LH patterns are often prepubertal or pubertal and show decreased, low-amplitude pulsations. The pattern of LH secretion can be artificially returned to normal by the

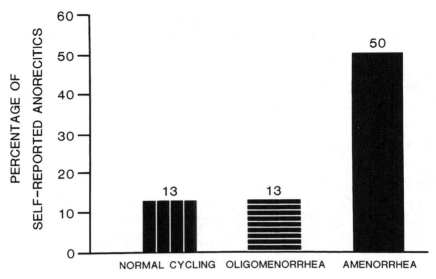

Figure 5.5 *Percentage of dancers with and without menstrual irregularities who reported anorexia nervosa. (Reproduced by permission from Brooks-Gunn J, Warren MP, Hamilton LH. The relation of eating problems and amenorrhea in ballet dancers. Med Sci Sports Exerc 1987;19:41–44, p. 43.)*

pulsatile administration of exogenous GnRH; follicular maturation, and even menstruation, can be induced in these severely hypoestrogenic patients. In addition to reproductive changes, a number of other abnormalities that suggest hypothalamic dysfunction have been described in anorexia nervosa: a deficiency in handling a water load thought to result from mild diabetes insipidus, abnormal thermoregulatory responses, and lack of shivering. Cortisol secretion appears to be altered with a higher 24-hour set point and occasionally a mild decrease in thyroid hormone T_3 (triiodo-thyronine); T_4 (thyroxine) is metabolized differently in this state, away from the formation of the active T_3 to the production of reverse T_3, an inactive metabolite.

Bulimics may also present menstrual irregularities, but reproductive dysfunction is not as severe, and these patients may be anovulatory with adequate estrogen secretion. Since this behavior is often secretive, and weight may remain within a normal range, a careful history and associated physical findings are important for the diagnosis. These include swollen parotid glands, tooth decay, cramps of the hands and feet (due to the development of a metabolic alkalosis secondary to vomiting), and the decrease in ionized calcium leading to tetanic seizures.

Another eating pattern of interest in young women is the trend toward vegetarian diets. This pattern is seen particularly in endurance athletes and in girls with highly restrictive diets. In patients with anorexia nervosa who have definite food preferences, the most frequent is vegetarianism. This pattern is important, in light of the fact that vegetarianism has recently been associated with a variety of hormonal abnormalities, and in general the American vegetarian diet has been found to be more nutrient- and calorie-deficient than nonvegetarian diets. The combination of vegetarian diets and overly restrictive dietary patterns and compulsive athletic activity may be a sign of poor psychological health and bears watching. The hormonal evaluation again requires tests of prolactin, LH, FSH, and possibly an estradiol. Progesterone in the form of medroxyprogesterone acetate can be given for 5 to 10 days to evaluate endogenous estrogen secretion.

Irregular Periods in Normal-Weight Athletes   If an eating disorder is ruled out, these individuals may fit into the category of athletes who have an anovulatory syndrome with increased LH levels. This syndrome has not been well studied. Evaluation should proceed as outlined above; the increased LH/FSH ratio will make the diagnosis. This group can be handled in the same way.

Management

Management of the Athlete with Menstrual Irregularities

Several factors must be considered, including the age of the athlete, her diet and caloric balance, the type of sport, the duration of the problem, the estrogen status, and her fertility intentions (pregnancy, contraception, and so on).

The most rational approach to an athlete's menstrual dysfunction is to reduce the amount of exercise or increase the caloric intake (if there is a negative caloric balance). A 10% decrease in exercise (either duration or intensity) or gain of 1 to 2 kg is recommended. However, the ideal energy balance for an athlete to maintain her menses without losing the artistic and athletic advantages of thinness is not yet known and probably varies from one athlete to another.

Management of the Athlete with Oligomenorrhea or Amenorrhea

After ruling out diseases, explanation and reassurance therapy should be started. Medroxyprogesterone, 10 mg for 5 to 10 days every month, will prevent the risk of endometrial hyperplasia and adenocarcinoma. If there is no withdrawal bleeding and if the athlete has low levels of Estradiol-17β (E_2), therapy to prevent osteoporosis should be given as discussed in Chapter 9. Oral contraceptives are a reasonable option if contraception is required, and clomiphene if pregnancy is desired.

Management of the Athlete with Short Luteal Phase

It seems that athletes with luteal phase deficiency do not require treatment unless they wish to conceive. Reduction or cessation of exercise will often reverse this condition, but many athletes prefer hormonal treatment over a change in lifestyle. These include progesterone suppositories, clomiphene citrate, or gonadotropin therapy. Calcium supplements are indicated, particularly because requirements range between 1000 and 1500 mg per day, and the athlete's diet is often deficient.

Management of Other Consequences of Menstrual Irregularity

Infertility may be a consequence of athletic activity and is reviewed in Chapter 9. Prolonged hypoestrogenism may cause a reversal of the beneficial change in plasma lipoprotein levels, although the consequences of these issues have not been well studied.

Bibliography

1. Brooks-Gunn J, Warren MP, Hamilton LH. The relation of eating problems and amenorrhea in ballet dancers. Med Sci Sports Exerc 1987;19:41–44.
2. Bullen BA, Skrinar GS, Beitins IZ, et al. Induction of menstrual disorders by strenuous exercise in untrained women. N Engl J Med 1985;312:1349–1353.
3. Cameron JL, Nosbisch C, Helmreich DL, Parfitt DB. Reversal of exercise-induced amenorrhea in female cynomolgus monkeys (Macaca Fascicularis) by increasing food intake. Endocrine Society Annual Meeting 1990;72:285. Abstract.

4. Constantini NW, Warren MP. Physical activity, fitness, and reproductive health in women: clinical observations. In: Bouchard C, Shephard RJ, Stephens T, eds. Physical activity, fitness, and health: international proceedings and consensus statement. Champaign, IL: Human Kinetics, 1994:955–966.

5. Constantini NW, Warren MP. Special problems of the female athlete. In: Panush RS, Lane NE, eds. Clinical rheumatology: exercise and rheumatic disease. London: Bailliere Tindall, 1994:199–219.

6. Constantini NW, Warren MP. Menstrual dysfunction in swimmers: a distinct entity. J Clin Endocrinol Metab, 1995;80:2740–2744.

7. DeSouza MJ, Metzger DA. Reproductive dysfunction in amenorrheic athletes and anorexic patients: a review. Med Sci Sports Exerc 1991;23:995–1007.

8. Gadpaille WJ, Sanborn CF, Wagner WW Jr. Athletic amenorrhea, major affective disorders, and eating disorders. Am J Psychiatry 1987;144:939–942.

9. Glass AR, Deuster PA, Kyle SB, et al. Amenorrhea in Olympic marathon runners. Fertil Steril 1987;48:740–745.

10. Highet R. Athletic amenorrhea: an update on aetiology, complications and management. Sports Med 1989;7:82–108.

11. Keizer HA, Rogol AD. Physical exercise and menstrual cycle alterations: what are the mechanisms? Sports Med 1990;10:218–235.

12. Loucks AB, Mortola JF, Girton L, Yen SSC. Alterations in the hypothalamic-pituitary-ovarian and the hypothalamic-pituitary-adrenal axes in athletic women. J Clin Endocrinol Metab 1989;68:402–411.

13. Loucks AB, Heath EM. Induction of low-T3 syndrome in exercising women occurs at a threshold of energy availability. Am J Physiol 1994;266:R817–R823.

14. Loucks AB, Brown R, King K, et al. A combined regimen of moderate dietary restriction and exercise training alters luteinizing hormone pulsatility in regularly menstruating young women. Endocrine Society Annual Meeting 1995;558.

15. Myerson M, Gutin B, Warren MP, et al. Resting metabolic rate and energy balance in amenorrheic and eumenorrheic runners. Med Sci Sports Exerc 1991;23:15–22.

16. Neinstein LS. Menstrual dysfunction in pathophysiologic states. Med 1985;143:476–484.

17. Prior JC, Ho Yuen B, Clement P, et al. Reversible luteal phase changes and infertility associated with marathon training. Lancet 1982;July:269–270.

18. Prior JC. Physical exercise and the neuroendocrine control of reproduction. Baillieres Clin Endocrinol Metab 1987;1:299–317.
19. Sanborn CF, Albrecht BH, Wagner WW Jr. Athletic amenorrhea: lack of association with body fat. Med Sci Sports Exerc 1987;19:207–212.
20. Warren MP. Reproductive disorders in dancers. In: Sataloff RT, Brandfonbrener A, Lederman R, eds. Textbook of performing arts medicine. New York: Raven, 1991:403–412.
21. Warren MP. Amenorrhea in endurance runners [Clinical Review 40]. J Clin Endocrinol Metab 1992;75:1393–1397.
22. Warren MP, Brooks-Gunn J. Delayed menarche in athletes: the role of low energy intake and eating disorders and their relation to bone density. In: Laron Z, Rogol AD, eds. Hormones and sport; vol. 55. New York: Serono Symposia Publications, 1989:41–54.
23. Warren MP, Brooks-Gunn J, Fox RP, et al. Lack of bone accretion and amenorrhea: evidence for a relative osteopenia in weight bearing bones. J Clin Endocrinol Metab 1991;72:847–853.
24. Warren MP, Brooks-Gunn J, Hamilton LH, et al. Scoliosis and fractures in young ballet dancers: relation to delayed menarche and secondary amenorrhea. N Engl J Med 1986;314:1348–1353.
25. Wilmore JH, Wambsgans KC, Brenner M, et al. Is there energy conservation in amenorrheic compared with eumenorrheic distance runners? J Appl Physiol 1992;72:15–22.
26. Wilson JS, Focimon C, Reyes FI, et al. Gonadotropins and steroid hormones in the blood and urine of prepubertal girls and other primates [Review]. J Clin Endocrinol Metabol 1978;7(3):513–530.
27. Yen SSC. Chronic anovulation due to CNS-hypothalamic-pituitary dysfunction. In: Yen SSC, Jaffe RB, eds. Reproductive endocrinology, 3rd. ed. Philadelphia: WB Saunders, 1991:631–688.

CHAPTER 6

The Adult Athlete: Dysmenorrhea

P rimary dysmenorrhea consists of pain accompanying the menstrual flow and is distinguishable from secondary dysmenorrhea by the absence of clearly identifiable pathology. The prevalence in the general population ranges from 47% to 80% in various age groups. This common disability usually appears during adolescence and tends to decrease with age and after pregnancy. It may cause significant absence from school and work, although most women experiencing dysmenorrhea (75% to 80%) report symptoms as mild, not severe. Symptoms include lower abdominal pain that may radiate to the lower back or legs, headache, nausea, and vomiting.

Biochemical evidence has linked the pathophysiology of primary dysmenorrhea to elevated levels of prostaglandins, which cause uterine contractions and ischemia. The role of prostaglandins has been indirectly confirmed by the effectiveness of prostaglandin inhibitors in reducing painful symptoms accompanying menstrual flow. Although increased prostaglandin levels have been reported in diverse studies of dysmenorrhea, the origin of this elevation remains a source of controversy. It has been most recently attributed to the fall of progesterone in the premenstrual phase, which, through a series of biochemical changes, results in initiation of the synthesis of prostaglandin in endometrial cells by membrane phospholipids. This would account for the effectiveness of oral contraceptives in ameliorating dysmenorrhea. Ovulation inhibition leads to endometrial hypoplasia, which in turn reduces the ability of the endometrium to synthesize prostaglandins. Dysmenorrhea has also been linked to deficient degradation of prostaglandin due to a defect in PGdehydrogenase, to the vasoconstrictive action of antidiuretic hormone (ADH), and to variations in the blood flow at the pelvic level, which may influence synthesis or breakdown of prostaglandin.

Exercise is generally thought to improve dysmenorrhea (see Figures 6.1 and 6.2). However, results of studies on the relationship between exercise or physical activity and dysmenorrhea are contradictory. Research in this area has been characterized by varying definitions of dysmenorrhea and activity, different modes of data collection, and disparate overall study design. Several studies have suggested that athletic activity of any type or level has a positive influence on menstrual symptoms, reducing pain and lowering negative mood states and negative affect not only during periods but throughout the cycle. Exercise has repeatedly been found to improve mood and decrease stress. This suggests that exercise may have only significantly improved mood and therefore lowered reports of dysmenorrhea, but not the actual physical symptoms. The results are further confounded by the failure to conceal the purpose of the study from the volunteers in many of the studies. Using volunteers who are not adequately blinded to the issue being researched has often been found to

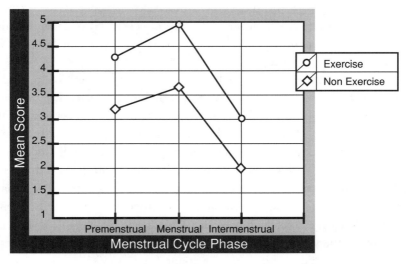

Figure 6.1 *Mean scores on psychological higher-order factor of Menstrual Distress Questionnaire. (Reproduced by permission of the publisher from Aganoff JA, Boyle GJ. Aerobic exercise, mood states and menstrual cycle symptoms. J Psychosom Res 1994;38:183–192, p. 186. Copyright 1994 by Elsevier Science Inc.)*

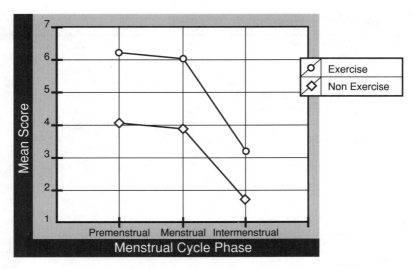

Figure 6.2 *Mean scores on physical higher-order factor of Menstrual Distress Questionnaire. (Reproduced by permission of the publisher from Aganoff JA, Boyle GJ. Aerobic exercise, mood states and menstrual cycle symptoms. J Psychosom Res 1994;38:183–192, p. 186. Copyright 1994 by Elsevier Science Inc.)*

introduce bias in studies that focus on the benefits of exercise. Furthermore, there is evidence that women report menstrual symptoms in a stereotypic manner when they believe these symptoms are of interest to the researcher.

In a study that did control for disposition and mood, Metheny and Smith (1989) reported that exercise is associated with higher levels of dysmenorrhea. The study was done on 176 student nurses, blind to the issue being researched, using a Menstrual Distress Questionnaire (see Table 6.1) and several other questionnaires designed to measure mood, disposition, exercise intensity, and perceived stress. Students who exercised regularly reported significantly lower levels of stress, had a more positive affect, and had a more optimistic outlook than sedentary students. After adjusting dysmenorrhea scores for disposition, perceived stress, mood, and medication, these exercising women showed an increase of 27% in menstrual symptom severity over nonexercising women. In addition, psychological stress was found to significantly affect reported levels of symptom severity, even after controlling for the other factors. Metheny and Smith suggest that although exercise relieves the stress that

Table 6.1 *Moos's menstrual distress questionnaire*

PLEASE COMPLETE THIS FORM EVERY EVENING TO DESCRIBE YOUR SYMPTOMS IN THE PREVIOUS 24 HOURS

On the page below is a list of symptoms which women sometimes experience. For each symptom choose the descriptive category listed below which best describes your experience of that symptom today. Circle the number of the category which best describes your experience of the symptom today. Even if none of the categories is exactly correct, choose the one that best describes your experience. Please be sure to circle one number for each symptom. Please also remember to put your name and the date in the blank spaces at the top of this page.

Descriptive   1. No reaction at all.   2. Barely noticeable.

Categories: 3. Present, mild.   4. Present, moderate.

5. Present, strong.   6. Acute, or partially disabling.

1. Weight gain	1	2	3	4	5	6
2. Insomnia	1	2	3	4	5	6
3. Crying	1	2	3	4	5	6
4. Lowered school or work performance	1	2	3	4	5	6
5. Muscle stiffness	1	2	3	4	5	6
6. Forgetfulness	1	2	3	4	5	6
7. Confusion	1	2	3	4	5	6
8. Take naps or stay in bed	1	2	3	4	5	6
9. Headache	1	2	3	4	5	6
10. Skin disorders	1	2	3	4	5	6
11. Loneliness	1	2	3	4	5	6
12. Feelings of suffocation	1	2	3	4	5	6
13. Affectionate	1	2	3	4	5	6
14. Orderliness	1	2	3	4	5	6
15. Stay at home from work or school	1	2	3	4	5	6
16. Cramps (uterine or pelvic)	1	2	3	4	5	6
17. Dizziness or faintness	1	2	3	4	5	6
18. Excitement	1	2	3	4	5	6
19. Chest pains	1	2	3	4	5	6
20. Avoid social activities	1	2	3	4	5	6
21. Anxiety	1	2	3	4	5	6
22. Backache	1	2	3	4	5	6

Table 6.1 *Continued*

23.	Cold sweats	1	2	3	4	5	6
24.	Lowered judgment	1	2	3	4	5	6
25.	Fatigue	1	2	3	4	5	6
26.	Nausea or vomiting	1	2	3	4	5	6
27.	Restlessness	1	2	3	4	5	6
28.	Hot flashes	1	2	3	4	5	6
29.	Difficulty in concentration	1	2	3	4	5	6
30.	Painful or tender breasts	1	2	3	4	5	6
31.	Feeling of well-being	1	2	3	4	5	6
32.	Buzzing or ringing in ears	1	2	3	4	5	6
33.	Distractable	1	2	3	4	5	6
34.	Swelling (e.g., abdomen, breasts, ankles)	1	2	3	4	5	6
35.	Accidents (e.g., cut finger, break dish)	1	2	3	4	5	6
36.	Irritability	1	2	3	4	5	6
37.	General aches and pains	1	2	3	4	5	6
38.	Mood swings	1	2	3	4	5	6
39.	Heart pounding	1	2	3	4	5	6
40.	Depression (feeling sad or blue)	1	2	3	4	5	6
41.	Decreased efficiency	1	2	3	4	5	6
42.	Lowered motor coordination	1	2	3	4	5	6
43.	Numbness or tingling in hands or feet	1	2	3	4	5	6
44.	Change in eating habits	1	2	3	4	5	6
45.	Tension	1	2	3	4	5	6
46.	Blind spots or fuzzy vision	1	2	3	4	5	6
47.	Bursts of energy or activity	1	2	3	4	5	6

Reproduced by permission from O'Brien PMS. Premenstrual syndrome. Oxford: Blackwell Science, 1987, p. 58.

may intensify dysmenorrhea, it may simultaneously aggravate these symptoms, perhaps by heightening somatic awareness. (Regular exercise has been associated with an increased sensitivity to bodily states.) Another possibility is that the exercising women reduced their activity levels during the premenstrual phase. This could result in a significant drop in endorphin levels, which might make menstrual pain seem more severe. The results of this study are confounded by the fact that menstrual cycle symptoms were reported retrospectively; this method has been shown to result in an exaggeration of responses compared with prospective reporting.

Other groups have found that exercise and physical activity have no effect on the occurrence of dysmenorrhea (see Table 6.2). Studies have focused on different age groups, from healthy adolescent girls to 415 residents of Singapore, aged 15 to 54. Several studies have examined

Table 6.2 *Prevalence of dysmenorrhea by selected risk factors*

Variable	n	Dysmenorrhea		p value
		Number	*Percentage*	
Age (years)				
≤30	174	115	66.1%	
>30	241	98	40.7%	<0.01
Age of menarche (years)				
≤12	148	89	60.1%	
>12	267	124	46.4%	<0.01
Parity (in married women)				
Nulliparous	29	17	58.6%	
Parous	236	95	40.3%	0.06
Physical activity				
Active	90	48	53.3%	
Inactive	325	165	50.8%	0.75
Smoking				
Current and ex-smokers	16	8	50.0%	
Nonsmokers	399	205	51.4%	0.91
Oral contraceptive usage				
User	19	12	63.2%	
Nonuser	396	201	50.8%	0.29

Reproduced by permission from Ng TP, Tan NCK, Wansaicheong GKL. A prevalence study of dysmenorrhoea in female residents aged 15–54 years in Clementi Town, Singapore. Ann Acad Med Singapore 1992;21:323–327, p. 325.

whether increasing the intensity or competitive level of exercise affects dysmenorrhea. Again, results are contradictory. One study found no difference in the incidence of dysmenorrhea between athletes engaging in hard physical activity and those engaging in moderate physical activity. This contradicts the results reported by Izzo and Labriola (1991), who found that women who exercise intensively report fewer dysmenorrhea symptoms than those who exercise only occasionally. Izzo and Labriola also found a difference in the type of symptoms reported. The intensive exercisers complained almost exclusively of backache and asthenia, while the nonintensive group reported a greater variability of symptoms, including irritability, general muscle pain, vomiting, and nausea.

Hata and Aoki (1990) studied Japanese athletes at four different competitive levels and found no association between higher levels of training and three of the four dysmenorrhea symptoms they studied. Nonathletes, high school athletes, college athletes, and young top athletes completed a questionnaire in which they were asked to recall whether they had experienced lower abdominal pain, headache, breastache, and backache. Higher levels of training correlated with a greater incidence of backache but not with any of the other three symptoms. The results could be confounded by the fact that dysmenorrhea has been shown to decrease with increasing age, and the exercising groups represent increasing age groups as well as increasing competitive levels.

The observed association between menstrual pain and absence from work has prompted many researchers to investigate the relationship between dysmenorrhea and working conditions. One study found an association between severe dysmenorrhea and shift work, particularly irregular shifts, in Japanese hospitals. Another study found a higher prevalence of dysmenorrhea in women working in Canadian slaughterhouses (73%) than in the wives of their male colleagues (57%). Menstrual pain was associated with exposure to cold, and increased cold exposure was associated with a greater percentage of absenteeism among dysmenorrheic workers.

In a similar study, Messing et al (1993) studied 726 women working in either slaughterhouses or canneries throughout western France. Women completed interviews and questionnaires that included questions about both living and working conditions and menstrual history. Dysmenorrhea was more prevalent among cannery workers than slaughterhouse workers. Messing et al attribute this disparity to differences in working conditions. Cannery workers more often reported exposure to cold temperatures, drafts, and high humidity, factors that were all associated with dysmenorrhea. In addition, women whose work required physical exertion, particularly lifting weights, were more likely to report dysmenorrhea. Messing et al point out that this association is not unexpected given the demands such work puts on the circulatory system. A strong relationship was also present between dysmenorrhea and a lack of freedom to leave the work position when necessary (for example, to go to the bathroom). General job satisfaction and number of working hours were not associated with pain, but no adjustment was made for psychological factors, such as mood and perceived stress. The high prevalence of dysmenorrhea among female workers points to the need for well-controlled studies in the future to further elucidate the relationship between menstrual pain and working conditions. Furthermore, the conflicting results of the effects of exercise on dysmenorrhea point to the need for carefully controlled longitudinal studies.

Bibliography

1. Aganoff JA, Boyle GJ. Aerobic exercise, mood states and menstrual cycle symptoms. J Psychosom Res 1994;38:183–192.
2. Anonymous. Premenstrual syndrome and dysmenorrhea. Baltimore: Urban and Schwarzenberg, 1985.
3. Aubuchon PG, Calhoun KS. Menstrual cycle symptomatology: the role of social expectancy and experimental demand characteristics. Psychosom Med 1985;47:35–45.
4. Boyle GJ, Grant AF. Prospective versus retrospective assessment of menstrual cycle symptoms and moods: role of attitudes and beliefs. J Psychopathology Behav Assess 1992;14:307–321.
5. Busch CM, Costa PT, Whitehead WE, Heller BR. Severe perimenstrual symptoms: prevalence and effects on absenteeism and health care seeking in a non-clinical sample. Women Health 1988;14:59–74.
6. Chan WY, Dawood MY, Fuchs F. Prostaglandins in primary dysmenorrhea. Comparison of prophylactic and nonprophylactic treatment with ibuprofen and use of oral contraceptives. Am J Med 1981;70:535–541.
7. Colt EW, Wardlaw SL, Frantz AG. The effect of running on plasma beta endorphin. Life Sci 1981;28:1637–1640.

8. Endicott J, Halbreich V. Retrospective report of premenstrual depressive changes: factors affecting confirmation by daily ratings. Psychopharmacol Bull 1982;48:109–112.

9. Folkins CH, Sime WE. Physical fitness training and mental health. American Psychol 1981;36:373–389.

10. Gannon L, Luchetta T, Pardie L, Rhodes K. Perimenstrual symptoms: relationships with chronic stress and selected lifestyle variables. J Behav Med 1989;15:149–159.

11. Hata E, Aoki K. Age at menarche and selected menstrual characteristics in young Japanese athletes. Research Quarterly for Exercise and Sport 1990;61:178–183.

12. Hughes JR. Psychological effects of habitual aerobic exercise: a critical review. Prev Med 1984;13:66–78.

13. Israel RG, Sutton M, O'Brien KF. Effects of aerobic training on primary dysmenorrhea symptomatology in college females. J Am Coll Health 1985;33:241–244.

14. Izzo A, Labriola D. Dysmenorroea and sports activities in adolescents. Clin Exp Obstet Gynecol 1991;18:109–116.

15. Martinsen EW. The role of aerobic exercise in the treatment of depression. Stress Med 1987;3:93–100.

16. Mergler D, Vezina N. Dysmenorrhea and cold exposure. J Reprod Med 1985;30:106–111.

17. Messing K, Saurel-Cubizolles M, Bourgine M, Kaminski M. Factors associated with dysmenorrhea among workers in French poultry slaughterhouses and canneries. J Occup Med 1993;35:493–500.

18. Metheny WP, Smith RP. The relationship among exercise, stress, and primary dysmenorrhea. J Behav Med 1989;12:569–586.

19. Morgan WP, Goldston SE. Exercise and mental health. New York: Hemisphere, 1987.

20. Ng TP, Tan NCK, Wansaicheong GKL. A prevalence study of dysmenorrhoea in female residents aged 15–54 years in Clementi Town, Singapore. Ann Acad Med Singapore 1992;21:323–327.

21. Parlee MB. Changes in moods and activation levels during the menstrual cycle in experimentally naive subjects. Psychology of Women Quarterly 1982;7:119–131.

22. Sultan C, Chotard AM, Sultan N, et al. Dysmenorrhée de l'adolescente. Rev Intern Pediatr 1984;138:25.

23. Sultan N, Sultan C, Pey R, Jean R. Variations of plasma 13–14 dihydro-15 ceto prostaglandins F2 in adolescent dysmenorrhoea. Pediatr Res 1984; 18:104.

24. Toriola AL, Mathur DN. Menstrual dysfunction in Nigerian athletes. Br J Obstet Gynaecol 1986;93:979–985.
25. Uehata T, Saskawa N. The fatigue and maternity disturbances of night work-women. J Hum Ergol (Tokyo) 1982;11(suppl):465–474.
26. Wilson C, Emans SJ, Mansfield J, et al. The relationships of calculated percent body fat, sports participation, age, and place of residence on menstrual patterns in healthy adolescent girls at an independent New England high school. J Adolesc Health Care 1984;5:248–253.

CHAPTER 7

The Adult Athlete: Premenstrual Syndrome

I n many women dysmenorrhea is preceded by premenstrual syndrome (PMS), which generally appears 2 to 10 days before menses begins. It has been reported that 58% of women who complain of dysmenorrhea also experience some premenstrual symptoms. Prevalence of PMS has been reported to range from 30% to 63% in populations of different ages, although there are reports that up to 97% of women experience at least some symptoms and mood changes premenstrually. For approximately 50% of women, the changes are minor, but for 35% the symptoms and mood alterations disrupt daily life, and for 5% to 10% the symptoms are severely debilitating. Analyzing prevalence studies and evaluating findings in premenstrual research is made more difficult by the frequent lack of clarity as to whether subjects fulfill the diagnostic criteria for actual PMS or are just experiencing some premenstrual symptoms. Clinical diagnosis of PMS requires a prospective self-report of at least one of six affective complaints (including depression, anxiety, and irritability) and at least one of four somatic complaints (breast tenderness, abdominal bloating, headache, and swelling of extremities) in at least two cycles. Identifiable dysfunction in social or economic performance by one of several criteria must also be present.

Although studies have repeatedly shown that exercise can lessen premenstrual emotional symptoms, data are contradictory as to whether physical symptoms are attenuated as well. In a retrospective study of 748 university students, Timonen and Procope (1971) found that physical education majors had fewer premenstrual emotional symptoms than their less active classmates but no significant difference in moliminal

57

symptoms. The type, intensity, and frequency of exercise was not documented. In contrast, Aganoff and Boyle (1994) recently found that regular, moderate, aerobic exercise has significant effects on both negative mood states and physical symptoms (pain, water retention, and autonomic reactions) across the entire menstrual cycle. Similar results have been previously reported by Prior et al (1986), Keye (1985), and Gannon et al (1989). Prior et al compared three groups: initially sedentary women who began running regularly, runners who increased their distances as part of marathon training, and nonexercising controls. The novice runners reported decreased breast tenderness, fluid retention, and stress, and the marathon runners reported less fluid retention, depression, and anxiety. The nonexercising controls showed no significant changes in premenstrual symptoms.

Aerobic exercise appears to have more beneficial effects on PMS than nonaerobic exercise. Steege and Blumenthal (1993) found that although both strength training and aerobic exercise were associated with a general improvement in premenstrual symptoms in middle-aged women, aerobic exercisers improved on more symptoms, particularly premenstrual depression. Twenty-three healthy premenopausal women, aged 45 to 55, were randomly assigned to either strength training or aerobic exercise. Fitness level and menstrual symptomatology (using a Menstrual Symptom Questionnaire) were assessed both at baseline and after three months. Premenstrual symptoms were more severe in these women than in the general population, a fact that the researchers attribute to the use of a retrospective reporting technique. Aerobic exercise was associated with more significant improvement on premenstrual depression, irritability, tension, concentration, and energy level. Although both groups showed an improvement of somatic symptoms, the strength trainers actually improved more significantly on bloating and abdominal heaviness. The results could have been confounded by the small sample size, the lack of a control group, and the failure to keep subjects adequately blinded to the research question.

In some cases premenstrual symptoms are sufficiently severe to cause absenteeism from work, so the association between working conditions and premenstrual syndrome has been investigated. In the study of French poultry and cannery workers mentioned in Chapter 6, pain before and during periods showed different relationships with working

Table 7.1   *Diagnostic criteria for late luteal phase dysphoric disorder*

1. For most menstrual cycles during the past year, symptoms in 2 occurred during the last week of the luteal phase and remitted within a few days after the onset of the follicular phase. In menstruating females this corresponds to the week prior to menses, and a few days after the onset of menses. In nonmenstruating females who have had a hysterectomy, the timing of luteal and follicular phases may require the measurement of circulating reproductive hormones.

2. At least five of the following symptoms were present for most of the time during each symptomatic periluteal phase; at least one of the symptoms was (a), (b), (c), or (d):

    a. Marked affective lability (e.g. suddenly sad, tearful, irritable, or angry)

    b. Persistent and marked anger or irritability

    c. Feeling extremely anxious, tense, keyed up, or on edge

    d. Markedly depressed mood, marked pessimism, or self-deprecating thoughts

    e. Decreased interest in usual activities (e.g. work, friends, hobbies)

    f. Easily tired or lack of energy

    g. Subjective sense of difficulty concentrating

    h. Marked change in appetite, overeating, or specific food cravings

    i. Hypersomnia or insomnia

    j. Other physical symptoms (e.g. breast tenderness or swelling, headaches, joint or muscle pain, sensation of "bloating," or weight gain)

3. The disturbance seriously interferes with work or with usual social activities or relationships with others.

4. The disturbance is not merely an exacerbation of the symptoms of another disorder, such as major depression, panic disorder, dysthymia, or a personality disorder, although it may be superimposed on any of these disorders.

5. Criteria 1, 2, 3, and 4 are confirmed by prospective daily self-ratings of at least two symptomatic cycles. The diagnosis may be made provisionally prior to this confirmation.

Source: American Psychiatric Association. Diagnostic and statistical manual of mental disorders, 3rd ed., rev. Washington, American Psychiatric Association, 1987. Reproduced by permission from Ferin M, Jewelewicz R, Warren MP. The menstrual cycle. New York: Oxford, 1993, p. 202.

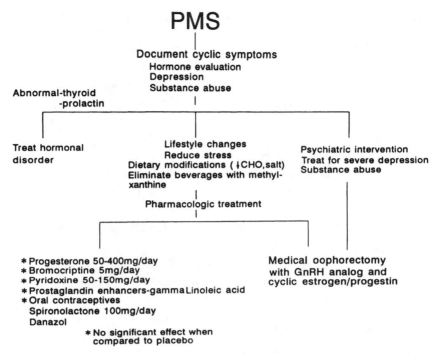

Figure 7.1   *General therapeutic outline for PMS. GnRH, gonadotropin-releasing hormone. (Reproduced by permission from Ferin M, Jewelewicz R, Warren MP. The menstrual cycle. New York: Oxford 1993, p. 203.)*

conditions. Premenstrual symptoms were associated with difficulty keeping up at work, with three or fewer breaks per day, and with an irregular workday beginning. No significant association was found with exposure to cold or with physical exertion, two factors that were related to dysmenorrhea.

The etiology of PMS has not been clearly defined despite the multitude of hypotheses that have been proposed. The disorder seems to be related to fluctuations in estrogen and progesterone, which may in turn be dependent on endorphin functioning. Estrogen's fluid-retaining action may lead to transient increases of fluid in different body tissues, which could explain symptoms such as weight gain, edema, breast tenderness, and bloating. Serotonin dysfunction, endogenous opioid withdrawal, and psychosomatic influences have not been ruled out as alternative hypotheses.

The physiologic explanation for the effects of exercise on menstrual symptoms remains unclear as well. It has been suggested that vigorous exercise acutely raises serum progesterone levels. These small increases, though insufficient to significantly alter the menstrual cycle, may alter mood by affecting neurotransmitter systems (for example, gamma-aminobutyric acid [GABA] and serotonin). Exercise may result in production of endorphins, which may improve mood. It may also simply provide psychological benefits by serving as a relief from the burdens of daily life or by improving body image and self-esteem.

Evaluation of the athlete with PMS will focus on an evaluation of problems as defined in the *Diagnostic and Statistical Manual of Mental Disorders* (see Table 7.1). Some of the symptoms may be present; the criteria has been criticized as lacking enough physical symptoms. A schema of treatment is outlined in Figure 7.1.

Bibliography

1. Aganoff JA, Boyle GJ. Aerobic exercise, mood states and menstrual cycle symptoms. J Psychosom Res 1994;38:183–192.
2. Gannon L, Luchetta T, Pardie L, Rhodes K. Perimenstrual symptoms: relationships with chronic stress and selected lifestyle variables. J Behav Med 1989;15:149–159.
3. Keye WR. Medical treatment of premenstrual syndrome. Can J Psychiatry 1985;30:483–487.
4. Messing K, Saurel-Cubizolles M, Bourgine M, Kaminski M. Factors associated with dysmenorrhea among workers in French poultry slaughterhouses and canneries. J Occup Med 1993;35:493–500.
5. O'Brien PMS. Premenstrual syndrome. Oxford: Blackwell Science, 1987.
6. Prior JC, Vigna Y, Alojado N. Conditioning exercise decreases premenstrual symptoms: a prospective controlled three month trial. Eur J Appl Physiol 1986;59:349–355.
7. Steege JF, Blumenthal JA. The effects of aerobic exercise on premenstrual symptoms in middle-aged women: a preliminary study. J Psychosom Res 1993;37:127–133.
8. Timonen S, Procope BJ. Premenstrual syndrome and physical exercise. Acta Obstet Gynecol Scand 1971;50:331–337.

9. Wilson C, Emans SJ, Mansfield J, et al. The relationships of calculated percent body fat, sports participation, age, and place of residence on menstrual patterns in healthy adolescent girls at an independent New England high school. J Adolesc Health Care 1984;5:248–253.
10. Woods NF, Most A, Dery GK. Prevalence of perimenstrual symptoms. Am J Public Health 1982;72:1257–1264.

The Adult Athlete: Other Gynecologic Problems

Physical Activity and Cancer

A sedentary lifestyle is known to increase the risk of colon cancer and has recently been associated with increased risks of breast and other gynecologic cancers. Although breast cancer is the most common form of cancer in women, occurring in one woman in nine, cancers of the reproductive tract account for approximately 13% of all malignancies and 10% of all cancer-related deaths in women in the United States. Data indicate that among women with confirmed reproductive tract cancers, almost 50% are diagnosed with endometrial cancer, 25% with ovarian cancer, 20% with cervical cancer, and less than 2% with vaginal cancer. Very few recent studies have investigated risk factors for cervical and vaginal cancer. Recent data on cancer of the breast, endometrium, and ovary reveal a number of shared risk factors, including age, age at menarche, nulliparity, low parity, and exogenous estrogen use.

Although there are several biologically plausible mechanisms through which physical activity could affect cancer risk, the exact pathway is unknown. Obesity is a known risk factor for cancer of the breast, endometrium, and ovary, and many researchers have proposed that any protective effect of exercise is derived from a reduction in weight and loss of body fat. Athletes have been shown to have as much as one-third less body fat than nonathletes even when their total body weights were comparable. Excess body fat facilitates the extraglandular conversion of androgen to more potent forms of estrogen compounds, which have been observed in women with breast cancer. Excess weight has also been associated with decreased capacity of serum globulin, which binds sex hormones. This could in turn lead to increased amounts of free serum estradiol, which may be related to both breast and endometrial cancer. Both exogenous estrogen use and increased endogenous estrogen exposure in women with polycystic ovarian disease or estrogen-producing tumors have been linked to endometrial cancer. In contrast, low body fat is associated with increased metabolism of estradiol to nonpotent 2-hydroxylated catechol estrogens. Furthermore, vigorous exercise delays menarche and frequently results in anovulation and an early onset of menopause. These conditions have been shown to reduce risks of cancer of the breast, endometrium, and ovary.

Dietary fat has often been associated with increased risks of breast and endometrial cancer. A relationship has also been observed between ovarian cancer and fat intake, although these data are somewhat contradictory. Athletic participation is frequently associated with a prudent diet and low fat intake, and low-fat diets have been shown to increase the metabolism of estrogen to nonpotent estrogens. Meat consumption has been shown to have an adverse effect on tumor development, possibly because of the use of estrogens in fattening livestock. In addition, the sodium nitrate commonly used as a meat preservative has been shown to combine with amines in the body to form nitrosamines, which are proven carcinogens in animals.

Other mechanisms not directly related to body fat might also come into play. For instance, exercise might boost the immune system against tumor growth, perhaps by reducing stress. Stress stimulates the production of cortisol, which may inhibit immune system functioning. In one study, a linkage was suggested between jogging, mood state, T-lymphocyte function, and the risk of carcinogenesis. On the other hand, physical exercise has also been shown to increase bowel motility and to decrease fecal transit time, which would reduce the absorption of sterol, an estrogen precursor that is excreted from the bile duct.

Despite the uncertainty as to the reason for the association, physical activity has repeatedly been found to exert a protective effect against cancer in women. Frisch et al (1992) reported that the lifetime occurrence rate of breast cancer and cancers of the reproductive system (uterus, ovary, cervix, and vagina) was significantly lower for women who participated in organized athletics in college than for their nonathletic class-mates. Alumnae of ten colleges completed a detailed questionnaire as part of a study designed to assess long-term health. Of the 5398 respondents, 2622 described themselves as former athletes and 2776 as former nonathletes. Athletes were defined as women who had been on at least one regularly practicing athletic team or who trained regularly on their own. The age-adjusted rates for reproductive tract cancers were 3.7 per thousand for athletes and 9.5 per thousand for nonathletes; for breast cancer the rates were 10.1 per thousand for athletes and 15.6 per thousand for nonathletes. Athletes also had a lower prevalence of benign tumors of both the reproductive tract and the breast, a finding that allows us to rule out a greater cancer mortality in general among athletes. And, since the prevalence rates for the nonathletic women are in accord with national data, it is unlikely that the reporting or selection technique confounded the results. Furthermore, the family histories of the athletes and nonathletes were similar, which makes it unlikely that genetic factors account for the disparity in prevalence rates.

Frisch et al observed a small but significant difference in relative body fat between athletes and nonathletes. Because the athletes began exercising at an earlier age than the nonathletes, this difference probably existed in the long term. This finding suggests that the protective effect of exercise is at least partially attributable to changes in body composition. Because the researchers did not control for potentially confounding factors, such as diet and weight history, however, it is not clear whether there is a benefit in exercise beyond the reduction in body fat. Given the many potential risk factors for malignancy, it is difficult to separate the effects of exercise per se from the effect of an active woman's physical composition, lifestyle, and diet. A fundamental problem is self-selection. Both athletes and workers in physically demanding occupations choose to involve themselves in physical activity, and a particular body build may be advantageous in certain sports or occupations. Similarly, obese women may gravitate to sedentary jobs. Furthermore, exercising and nonexercising women may exhibit different health behaviors. Exercise has often been linked to other positive health practices, such as breast self-examination. On the other hand, it has also been reported that women who exercise regularly are less informed about breast cancer and practice self-examination less regularly than sedentary women, perhaps because they believe that exercise makes them less susceptible to cancer. Finally, a woman who exercises or holds a physically demanding job may have been exposed to many other lifestyle factors that could influence the association, such as a low fat–high fiber diet and stress-reducing activities.

Even moderate physical activity has been shown to afford protection from breast and gynecologic cancers. In a study conducted in Shanghai, Zheng et al (1993) linked employment data for 3783 cancer patients with occupational census data. The incidence of cancer of the breast, endometrium, and ovary was elevated in women whose jobs involved low energy expenditure and long sitting time, and was reduced among women with high-activity jobs. This trend was particularly pronounced for breast cancer. Since Zheng et al did not adjust for body fat, diet, number of pregnancies, or age at first birth, it is impossible to pinpoint the reason for the decreased cancer incidence and difficult to eliminate the confounding influence of socioeconomic status. The incidence of breast cancer was significantly higher for professionals, government officials, and clerical workers and was lower for service workers and craftsmen. The same general trends were observed for endometrial and ovarian cancer, although the associations were not statistically significant. In China, women in white-collar occupations are generally better educated and are therefore more likely to adopt Western lifestyles and diet, including a high fat intake. Low parity and age at first birth could also be related to socioeconomic status. Although the study's findings are significant, it may be that other factors aside from activity account for the decreased incidence of cancer among more active women.

In a study of Finnish female teachers, Pukkala et al (1993) reported a slight difference in total cancer risk between active and nonactive women, but they found that the association between activity and reduced incidence was not strong enough to eliminate the confounding effect of high socioeconomic status. Only in the case of breast cancer did physical activity exert a significant protective effect, and this was evident only in premenopausal women. A total of 1499 physical education teachers and 8619 language teachers were identified from registers. When a questionnaire was given to a random sample of these teachers to identify any confounding differences between the two groups, clear disparities were present in estimates of physical activity, but there were no significant differences in body mass index, dietary fat intake, lifestyle estimates, and gynecologic risk factors. The incidence of reproductive system cancers did not differ significantly between groups in the entire sample, but the incidence of cancer in both groups was slightly higher than the average for the Finnish population. The researchers suggest that this finding may be attributable to the teachers' slightly higher social status. In Finland, working-age women belonging to higher social classes have been found to demonstrate a significantly elevated risk for breast cancer and a slightly elevated risk for endometrial and ovarian cancer. Despite the apparent importance of controlling for socioeconomic status, the researchers used only a subgroup to assess whether the entire subject population differed on any of the potential confounding factors. It could be that the surveyed group was not a sufficiently representative socioeconomic sample. Furthermore, Pukkala et al found that even the language teachers were more active than average Finnish women. Perhaps a larger contrast in activity levels between subgroups would allow for more effective evaluation of cancer risk in active and nonactive women.

Several studies that control for body weight and diet have specifically investigated the relationship between activity and endometrial cancer. Studies of endometrial cancer may be less problematic than studies of other cancers, since it is commonly detected at an earlier stage. This reduces the likelihood that lower activity reflects a change in response to preclinical illness. Sturgeon et al (1993) found that inactivity was associated with an increased incidence of endometrial cancer. Sustained inactivity in particular was similarly associated with increased risk. Cases were 20- to 74-year-old residents in defined geographic regions with confirmed incident endometrial cancer, and matched controls were women contacted through random digit-dialing techniques. Subjects were asked questions pertaining to known risk factors, such as diet and pregnancy history, as well as objective and subjective questions about lifetime physical activity. Interestingly, nonrecreational activity was associated with an increase in endometrial cancer risk, even after adjusting for excess body mass. This finding suggests that physical inactivity may influence cancer risk through a mechanism that does not directly involve obesity. Similarly, for recreational activity, an association between inactivity and risk persisted after taking body mass into account, but in this case, the association was found only in overweight women. This suggests that the study did not fully control for unmeasured lifestyle factors related to obesity. Since endometrial cancer is directly related to obesity, it is important to eliminate this factor in such a study. Data could also have been confounded by the fact that an active heavy woman and an inactive heavy woman may have the same body mass but different percentages of body fat.

In a population-based study conducted in China, Shu et al (1993) similarly found that women who hold sedentary jobs or report sedentary lifestyles are at a higher risk for endometrial cancer than more active women. All 18- to 70-year-old women diagnosed with endometrial cancer in an eighteen-month period were identified from the Shanghai Cancer Registry. The 258 cases and age-matched controls completed an interview that included a self-rating of past and present physical activity levels as well as objective questions about physical activity both inside and outside of work. Even after adjusting for number of pregnancies, age, body mass index, and caloric intake, Shu et al found that sedentary jobs were related to an increased risk of endometrial cancer. This association was, however, restricted to nonretired women. For women over age 55, the average retirement age in the study, sedentary jobs were actually related to reduced risks of endometrial cancer. This could suggest that occupational physical activity is not an accurate indicator of physical activity among retired women. It could also be related to the fact that endometrial cancer is known to be a disease that predominantly occurs in postmenopausal women; the peak incidence is at 58 to 60 years. These results, though, contradict data collected by Zheng et al, who found that the inverse association of cancer risk with occupational physical activity was stronger in retired women.

In a case-controlled study conducted in Switzerland and Italy, Levi et al (1993) found that moderate or high physical activity is an indicator of reduced endometrial cancer risk among women of all ages, both retired and nonretired. Women with histologically confirmed endometrial cancer were compared with hospital patients whose primary diagnosis was unrelated to any of the known or potential risk factors for endometrial cancer. Structured interviews included both objective and subjective measures of physical activity. Even after allowances were made for body mass index and caloric intake, subjects tended to report more frequently "low" or "very low" physical activity. The relative risks were similar for "moderately high" or "very high" physical activity. Housework, sports and leisure activities, and occupational activity were significantly associated with endometrial cancer risk, although no association was observed for climbing stairs or walking. The fact that the association was strongest for housework and sports and leisure activities suggests that lifestyle factors or socioeconomic status could at least partially account for the change in cancer incidence.

As American women continue to see improved longevity, the incidence of reproductive tract cancers is expected to increase proportionately. Though data are not conclusive, evidence suggests that exercise may result in long-term protection from breast and some reproductive cancers. This underscores the importance of continuing to investigate how physical activity in itself affects cancer incidence. Future studies should include measurements of body fat and detailed assessments of physical activity, including intensity and duration, and should aim to control for many potentially confounding lifestyle factors.

Urinary Incontinence

Though involuntary urine loss has usually been regarded as a problem restricted to older, multiparous women, studies have repeatedly shown that it occurs fairly commonly in younger, highly fit, nulliparous women as well. Several researchers have found that about 40% of young women have experienced urinary incontinence at least once, and about 15% experience it at least occasionally during daily life.

Exercise with high impact results in more episodes of incontinence. Bo et al (1989) studied the occurrence of involuntary urine loss in both sedentary nutrition students and physical education students exercising more than three times a week. They found a greater prevalence of urinary incontinence among the exercising physical education students (31% versus 10%). Differences were due to the occurrence of urine loss associated with jumping and running in the exercising women and were not significant when coughing, sneezing, or laughing were compared.

Nygaard and coworkers have conducted several studies in which they found that high-impact activities are likely to provoke urinary incontinence. Nulliparous college varsity athletes completed a questionnaire about the occurrence of urinary incontinence during their sports activities and during daily life. On average, 28% reported urine loss while participating in their sport. Combining the results of their studies, the incidence was greater for women in gymnastics, high-impact aerobics, running, and tennis than for those in swimming, weight-lifting, and golf. Athletes who noticed incontinence during sports were more likely to notice urine loss during daily life. Incontinence was not related to menstrual regularity, height, weight, or duration of playing time.

High-impact sports create a greater increase in intra-abdominal force than other athletic activities. Nygaard et al (1994) suggest that there is a continence threshold, a point beyond which a normally continent woman will become temporarily incontinent because of the increase in biomechanical forces. Pelvic muscles must be able to contract forcefully to withstand the weight of the abdominal viscera landing on the pelvic floor during repetitive jumping or running. Incontinence has been shown to occur when the pelvic floor has been exposed to more than a certain level of stress, or possibly when it is fatigued by general exercise. By wearing protective footwear or landing on the balls of their feet, athletes may minimize the occurrence of incontinence by lessening the amount of pressure that is transmitted to the pelvic floor. Pelvic muscle exercises, called Kegel exercises, are used as a behavioral treatment for incontinence.

Changes in connective tissue or collagen may be another factor involved in the failure of continence mechanisms. A properly functioning pelvic floor, among other things, provides support for pelvic viscera through a group of structures including connective tissue, muscles, and bones. Research has not yet shown whether exercise strengthens pelvic muscles as overall muscle fitness improves, or weakens pelvic muscles and connective tissue because of increases in intra-abdominal pressure. In one study, nulliparous women with stress incontinence were found to have a reduction in tissue collagen concentration compared to continent controls. Weakened connective tissue could lead to descent of the pelvic organ from its normal position, a condition known as genital prolapse.

Bibliography

Physical Activity and Cancer

1. Averette HE, Steren A, Nguyen HN. Screening in gynecologic cancer. Cancer 1993;72:1043–1049.

2. Blair SN, Jacobs DR, Powell KE. Relationships between exercise or physical activity and other health behaviors. Public Health Rep 1985;100:172–180.

3. Frisch RE, Wyshak G, Albright NL, et al. Former athletes have a lower lifetime occurrence of breast cancer and cancers of the reproductive system. In: Jacobs MM, ed. Exercise, calories, fat and cancer. New York: Plenum, 1992:29–39.

4. Gerard EL, Snow RC, Kennedy DN, et al. Overall body fat and regional fat distribution in young women: quantification with MR imaging. AJR Am J Roentgenol 1991;157:99–104.

5. Holdstock DJ, Misiewicz JJ, Smith T, Rowlands EN. Propulsion (mass movements) in the human colon and its relationship to meals and somatic activity. Gut 1970;11:91–99.

6. Kelsey JL, Berkowitz GS. Breast cancer epidemiology. Cancer Res 1988;48:5615–5623.

7. Levi F, La Vecchia C, Negri E, Franceschi S. Selected physical activities and the risk of endometrial cancer. Br J Cancer 1993;67:846–851.

8. MacKinnon LT, Chick TW, VanAs A, Tomasi TB. Effects of prolonged intense exercise on natural killer cells. Med Sci Sports Exerc 1987;19(suppl):S10.

9. Parazzini F, Franceschi S, La Vecchia C, Fasoli M. The epidemiology of ovarian cancer. Gynecol Oncol 1991;43:9–23.

10. Parazzini F, La Vecchia C, Bocciolone L, Franceschi S. The epidemiology of endometrial cancer. Gynecol Oncol 1991;41:1–16.

11. Platz CE, Benda J. Female genital tract cancer. Cancer 1995;75:270–294.

12. Pukkala E, Poskiparta M, Apter D, Vihko V. Life-long physical activity and cancer risk among Finnish female teachers. European Journal of Cancer Prevention 1993;2:369–376.

13. Rimpela AH, Pukkala EI. Cancers of affluence: positive social class gradient and rising incidence trend in some cancer forms. Soc Sci Med 1987;24:601–606.

14. Schlueter LA. Knowledge and beliefs about breast cancer and breast self-examination among athletic and nonathletic women. Nurs Res 1982;31:348–353.

15. Schneider JD, Kinne A, Fracchia A. Abnormal oxidative metabolism of estradiol in women with breast cancer. Proc Natl Acad Sci U S A 1982;79:3047–3051.
16. Shephard RJ. Exercise and malignancy. Sports Med 1986;3:235–241.
17. Shu XO, Hatch MC, Zheng W, et al. Physical activity and risk of endometrial cancer. Epidemiology 1993;4:342–349.
18. Simonton C. Jogging and cancer. Medicine and Sport 1978;12:124–125.
19. Sturgeon SR, Brinton LA, Berman ML, et al. Past and present physical activity and endometrial cancer risk. Br J Cancer 1993;68:584–589.
20. Turnbull EM. Effects of basic preventive health practices and mass media on the practice of breast self-examination. Nurs Res 1978;27:98–102.
21. Zheng W, Shu XO, McLaughlin JK, et al. Occupational physical activity and the incidence of cancer of the breast, corpus uteri, and ovary in Shanghai. Cancer 1993;71:3620–3624.

Urinary Incontinence

1. Bo K, Maehlum S, Oseid S, Larsen S. Prevalence of stress urinary incontinence among physically active and sedentary female students. Scand J Sports Sci 1989;11:113–116.
2. Nemir A, Middleton RP. Stress incontinence in young nulliparous women. Am J Obstet Gynecol 1954;68:1166–1168.
3. Nygaard IE, DeLancey JO, Arnsdorf L, Murphy E. Exercise and incontinence. Obstet Gynecol 1990;75:848–851.
4. Nygaard IE, Thompson FL, Svengalis SL, Albright JP. Urinary incontinence in elite nulliparous athletes. Obstet Gynecol 1994;84:183–187.
5. Wolin LH. Stress incontinence in young, healthy nulliparous female subjects. J Urol 1969;101:545–549.

CHAPTER 9

The Adult Athlete: Complications of Reproductive Problems

Infertility

Exercise and Infertility

Exercising women may experience infertility not only if they are amenorrheic or oligomenorrheic but also if they menstruate regularly but have luteal phase defects. Alterations in the menstrual cycle that lead to infertility may be the body's strategy to conserve energy for more essential biological functions. Apparently no published studies have examined the prevalence of exercise-induced infertility or the specific relationship between exercise and infertility. Researching the incidence of infertility among athletes is complicated by the fact that many women who menstruate regularly are not aware that they are experiencing anovulation or shortened luteal phase until they attempt to conceive.

Ovulatory disturbances have been repeatedly documented in exercising women. Alterations appear to be related not to the exercise itself but to training or exercise intensification. Early studies of rats showed that impaired follicle development occurs with abrupt increases in exercise but that normal reproductive function is maintained when the increase in exercise is gradual. Prior et al (1991) similarly found that in women, ovulatory changes occur in response to higher levels of training (see Figure 9.1) but return to normal when exercise reaches a steady level. It is likely that exercise leads to alterations in the GnRH pulse generator, but it is unclear exactly what produces these changes. One possibility is that the hypothalamus registers the low insulin levels or high core temperature levels that occur with training. Or, perhaps sensors in the hypothalamus

73

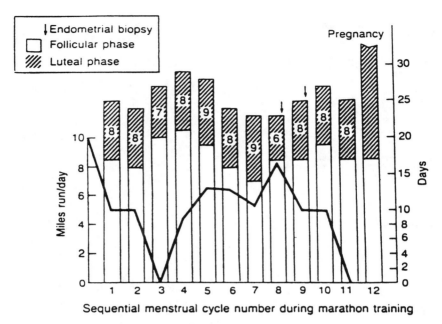

Figure 9.1 *Menstrual cycle phases in 12 consecutive cycles and number of miles run daily. The entire bar represents cycle length, the crosshatched area luteal length in days. Daily mileage is shown in the line graph at the bottom. (Reproduced by permission from Prior JC, Ho Yuen B, Clement P, et al. Reversible luteal phase changes and infertility associated with marathon training. Lancet 1982;11:269–270, p. 270. © by The Lancet Ltd. 1982.)*

detect changes in neurotransmitter input from the limbic system or hormonal changes that occur during emotional stress.

Though exercise probably exerts an important effect, it may not lead to menstrual cycle disturbances in the absence of other factors such as low body weight, weight loss, eating disorders, and perceived stress. Studies relating exercise to ovulatory disturbances have generally not controlled other factors associated with reproductive dysfunction. Body fat changes are no longer believed to be the critical event leading to menstrual irregularity and consequently to infertility, but they probably play an important role, particularly if frequent fluctuation releases metabolic signals affecting hypothalamic function. Exercise and weight loss seem to have an additive effect on menstrual disturbances. In a study of college-aged women, women were divided into weight loss and maintenance groups, and their estrogen and progesterone levels were measured daily through two cycles of increasing exercise and one control cycle. The groups had a similar incidence of abnormal luteal function, but in the weight loss group there was a progression from shortened luteal phase to anovulation. Furthermore, stress appears to be related to ovulatory disturbances even in the absence of weight loss and exercise. In one study, a group of sedentary women who ran as part of an experiment had a higher incidence of luteal phase defects than the runners with whom they were compared (29% versus 17%). The researchers attribute this to the greater perception of stress in the sedentary women.

Luteal phase defects and the resulting loss of fertility appear to be reversible in women who exercise or practice dietary restriction. Prior et al (1982) observed that in one marathon trainer, the luteal phase lengthened to 13 days after the race was complete and normal exercise was resumed. Another woman with a short luteal phase became pregnant 6 weeks after stopping intense running. Though this finding is significant, the failure to record changes in dietary intake makes it impossible to pinpoint decreased exercise as the reason for the resumed fertility. Bates et al (1982) found that infertility in women practicing dietary restriction is reversible. The researchers studied 29 women with unexplained infertility, 83% of whom were unaware of their menstrual dysfunction (either anovulatory cycles or a shortened luteal phase). Women were encouraged to gain weight to reach their ideal body weight (IBW) as defined by the Metropolitan Life Insurance Height and Weight Table. Of the 29 women, 26 were able to reach 98% of their IBW, and the resulting rate of successful pregnancy among those 26 women was 73%. When body weight approached IBW, a normal LH/FSH ratio was restored and menstrual cycles resumed normal ovulatory function (see Figure 9.2).

The incidence of infertility is high and continually increasing. The difficulty in isolating the impact of exercise on reproductive function from the effects of weight loss, stress, and other factors underscores the need for further carefully designed studies.

Evaluation of Women with Infertility

These patients should have a complete history and physical and the appropriate hormonal testing if they suffer from menstrual irregularity

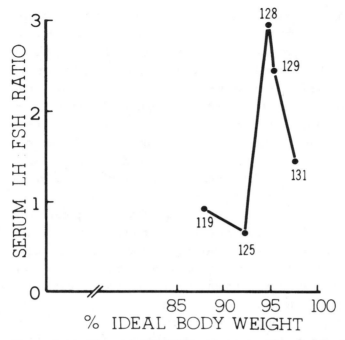

Figure 9.2 *Changing LH/FSH ratios in a 68-inch-tall, slender, infertile woman. Note the rise and fall in the LH/FSH ratio as she gained weight. She conceived at 131 pounds. (Reproduced by permission from Bates GW. Body weight control practice as a cause of infertility. Clin Obstet Gynecol 1985;28:632–663, p. 656.)*

and amenorrhea. A careful history should be taken regarding weight loss and excessive exercise, since hormonal changes may be subtle in women with inadequate luteal phases. A full evaluation for infertility is indicated, however, including semen analysis, postcoital test, endometrial biopsy, and most often hysterosalpingogram. Occasionally, a woman with amenorrhea may prefer to cut down on exercise or gain weight to see if normal cycles return. An athlete will very often resume menses within a few months provided the problem is of short duration (6 months or less) and is not associated with severe weight loss or anorexia nervosa.

Treatment of Women with Infertility

Weight gain (to at least 90% of IBW) and a decrease in exercise may be sufficient to treat ovulatory dysfunction. If more aggressive treatment is needed, induction of ovulation is accomplished by traditional means. These patients are often hypoestrogenic and do not respond to clomiphene citrate, but they may respond well to FSH and LH (Pergonal). Clomiphene should be tried first, however, and hCG can often be added when follicular maturation occurs to trigger ovulation. Cyclic menstrual function can also be restored in weight-related hypothalamic amenorrhea by means of pulsatile administration of GnRH administered with the aid of a pump by the subcutaneous or intravenous route.

Osteoporosis and Injury

Osteoporosis and skeletal problems have been reported in hypoestrogenic amenorrheic athletes. The loss of bone mass and lack of bone accretion seen in young amenorrheic athletes, in other amenorrheic groups, and recently in groups with delayed menarche and delayed development are potential hazards to both immediate and long-term health. In adolescents, scoliosis has been reported in ballet dancers with alarming frequency (up to 30%) and is directly related to a delay in the first period (see Figure 9.3). Osteopenia, particularly of trabecular bones, is common, and the rate of bone loss is similar to that associated with menopause: 5% per year. Injuries such as stress fractures and femoral head collapse may be due to weakened bone exposure to the impact of exercise, particularly with overuse syndromes. Recent evidence strongly suggests that young patients may also not be attaining their peak mass and that the osteopenia is due to lack of bone accretion rather than bone loss. Bone mass accumulation may continue until the early 30s, but this process may not progress normally in the absence of estrogen.

Stress or other fractures in an athlete who has hypoestrogenic amenorrhea may be an indication for treatment, particularly when a change in lifestyle (such as weight gain or a decrease in exercise) is not feasible or is rejected by the patient. Past research has focused on bone loss in postmenopausal women, but peak bone mass may be an equally important determinant of future osteoporosis and fractures. Studies have suggested that the incidence of stress fractures, scoliosis, vertebral compression fractures, and femoral head collapse observed in young women may be related to bone that is weakened by subjection to the stress of weight-bearing exercise. These injuries may be similar to those seen in hypoestrogenic postmenopausal women. The decrease in bone mass may

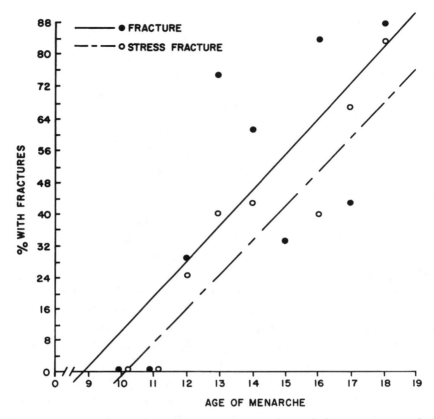

Figure 9.3   *Relation between age at menarche and the percentage of dancers with fractures (r = 0.68) and stress fractures (r = 0.63) (n = 75). (Reproduced by permission from Warren MP, Brooks-Gunn J, Hamilton LH, et al. Scoliosis and fractures in young ballet dancers: relation to delayed menarche and secondary amenorrhea. N Engl J Med 1986;314:1348–1353, p. 1351. Copyright 1986 Massachusetts Medical Society. All rights reserved.)*

also be irreversible. Our studies in young dancers suggest that increases in bone mass do occur in young individuals, even prior to return of normal menses, but still remain below normal despite these increases. Bone mass has not reversed with therapy in the dosages used, possibly because of prolonged hypoestrogenism in adolescence. There is great need for clinical trials to demonstrate the benefit of exogenous estrogen in this age group. Estrogen therapy and oral contraceptives continue to be used, however, as treatment in young women with amenorrhea. Recent work suggests that normal women who use oral contraceptives may have higher bone mass. One study reports that medical castration with GnRH and oral contraceptives had no effect on bone; another study shows that in the GnRH-treated women, the standard 0.625-mg dose of estrogen (Premarin) is not sufficient to protect against bone loss but that a doubling of the dose to 1.25 mg does give protection. This suggests that, in the hypogonadal model, a higher dose is necessary to maintain bone mass than in older women.

Bone mass formation increases dramatically at puberty (up to 40%), and past studies have shown that increases continue until age 34—although recent studies suggest no increase after age 20. Other studies have reported a decrease in bone mineral density (BMD) as early as age 20, while still others show no loss until age 44. Factors affecting peak bone mass include weight, body surface area, body mass, physical activity, calcium intake, genetics, and estrogen exposure. Studies suggest that women under age 30 have potential for increasing bone mass. Lack of bone mass is associated with significant clinical problems; young amenorrheic female athletes show a significantly higher injury rate (see Table 9.1).

There has been recent interest in the reversal of amenorrhea and its effect on bone density. Some studies have shown little or no reversal;

Table 9.1   *Incidence of stress fractures in amenorrheic and eumenorrheic athletes*

Reference	Sport	Amenorrheic (Number of Athletes)	Eumenorrheic (Number of Athletes)
Lindberg et al (1984)	Runners	49% (11)	0% (15)
Warren (unpublished)	Dancers[a]	65% (20)	25% (20)
Lloyd et al (1986)	Mixed	15% (41)	4% (158)
Barrow and Saha (1988)	Runners	49% (69)	29% (120)
Marcus et al (1985)	Runners	55% (11)	17% (6)
Clark et al (1988)	Runners	72% (18)	36% (75)

[a] Professional ballet dancers
Reproduced by permission from Constantini NW. Clinical consequences of athletic amenorrhea. Sports Medicine 1994;17:213–223, p. 218.

others have suggested that increases occur prior to reversal of the hypogonadal state. Therapy with estrogen replacement has been of great interest. Several authors have suggested that estrogen may have an independent effect on bone mass and that weight gain in particular may affect bone mass in a separate manner. No long-term study on estrogen replacement has been reported, although a number of cross-sectional studies suggest that in the pure hypogonadal state, estrogen therapy may be effective. Preliminary studies on small numbers of subjects ($n = 4$) suggest that oral contraceptives may be effective in athletic amenorrhea, although a recent report that included subjects on estrogens and oral contraceptives indicated no effect resulting from the contraceptives. Others have suggested that the hypercortisolemia seen in anorexia nervosa and athletically induced amenorrhea are related to the osteopenia. Alternatively, the estrogen dosages used to replace adolescent hypoestrogenism in some studies may be less than optimal to compensate for the rapid increase in bone density that occurs during puberty. One study that specifically examined estrogen replacement in adolescents and young adults noted lowered BMD in this group, despite estrogen. This study suggested that daily and possibly higher levels of estrogen replacement may be needed for adolescents and that unidentified factors may be responsible for the poor outcome in estrogen-deficient patients.

The triad of amenorrhea, osteopenia, and eating disorders in the female athlete has been the source of much publicity. The mechanism by which caloric restriction and abnormal eating may compromise bone mass is unclear. Multiple factors are affected by dietary restriction in hypothalamic amenorrhea, including depression of thyroid hormones and growth hormone. T_3 is a powerful and a potent stimulator of bone turnover, and GH is known to have stimulatory effects on bone formation in vivo and is necessary for maintenance of normal bone mass. GH is thought to stimulate insulin-like growth factor 1 (IGF1) by skeletal cells and, through this local factor, may regulate bone formation. These multiple processes of bone metabolism may be affected in the nutritionally restricted model.

Estrogen is given cyclically in combination with a progestin. Premarin or its equivalent is given in doses of 0.625 mg for 25 days, with 10 mg of Provera added on days 17 to 25. A week without therapy follows. This dose is thought to be protective for the bones, and a patient may or may not have cyclic bleeding. If periods are desired, the patient may need to take 1.25–2.5 mg of Premarin, or its equivalent, each day. Patients who have been hypoestrogenic for longer than a year will need 5 mg of Premarin to stimulate a very underactive endometrium. Recent studies suggest that estrogen in replacement doses may not be sufficient to protect against bone loss or to encourage bone accretion. Larger doses, or alternatively, oral contraceptives that provide 3 to 4 times replacement doses,

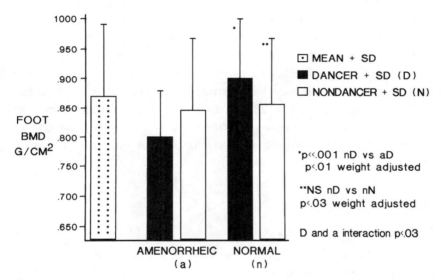

Figure 9.4 *Foot bone mineral densities in normal and amenorrheic subjects. Groups are divided into dancers and nondancers. Significance determined by analysis of variance, P < 0.05. The stippled bar represents the mean of all values. Two-way analysis of variance shows a significant effect of amenorrhea on bone mineral density even when controlling for age but was eliminated by controlling for weight. (Reproduced by permission from Warren MP, Brooks-Gunn J, Fox RP, et al. Lack of bone accretion and amenorrhea: evidence for a relative osteopenia in weight-bearing bones. J Clin Endocrinol Metab 1991;72:847–853, p. 850. © The Endocrine Society.)*
Multiple comparisons show that amenorrheic dancers differ from normal dancers even when controlling for age and weight.
**Normal dancers were higher than both amenorrheic groups when controlling for age. Interaction eliminated when controlling for age but not weight.*

may be needed. Work needs to be done to determine the factors that cause the osteopenia in the athlete.

Subjects who have not completed their growth should not receive hormones because of the risk of epiphyseal closure. Growth potential may be determined by a bone age study.

Exercise has also been recommended to preserve or increase bone mass. The effect is very small but appears to be beneficial, particularly in the postmenopausal population. However, recent data suggest that young hypoestrogenic ballet dancers may not accumulate bone in response to mechanical stress (see Figure 9.4). This observation stands in contrast to the mature, postmenopausal women in whom exercise will offset the loss seen with hypoestrogenism; in some cases postmenopausal women may experience an increase over baseline. These observations raise an issue that has not been well addressed: Should the young athlete who has not reached peak bone mass because of a delay in sexual development have activity curtailed to prevent stress fractures and other injuries due to overuse? The answer to this question is not clearcut and warrants further research.

Bibliography

Infertility

1. Bates GW. Body weight control practice as a cause of infertility. Clin Obstet Gynecol 1985;28:632–644.
2. Bates GW, Bates SR, Whitworth NS. Reproductive failure in women who practice weight control. Fertil Steril 1982;37:373–378.
3. Bullen BA, Skrinar GS, Beitins IZ, et al. Induction of menstrual disorders by strenuous exercise in untrained women. N Engl J Med 1985;312:1349–1353.
4. Prior JC. Endocrine "conditioning" with endurance training: a preliminary review. Can J Sport Sci 1982;7:148–156.
5. Prior JC, Vigna YM. Gonadal steroids in athletic women. Sports Med 1985;2:287–295.
6. Prior JC, Vigna YM. Ovulation disturbances and exercise training. Clin Obstet Gynecol 1991;34:180–190.

Osteoporosis and Injury

1. Ayers JW, Gidwani GP, Schmidt IM, Gross M. Osteopenia in hypoestrogenic women with anorexia nervosa. Fertil Steril 1984;41:224–228.

2. Barrow GW, Saha S. Menstrual irregularity and stress fractures in collegiate female distance runners. Am J Sports Med 1988;16:209–216.

3. Biller BMK, Saxe V, Herzog DB, et al. Mechanisms of osteoporosis in adult and adolescent women with anorexia nervosa. J Clin Endocrinol Metab 1989;68:548–554.

4. Biller BMK, Schoenfeld D, Klibanski A. Premenopausal osteopenia: effects of estrogen administration (#1616). Endocrine Society Annual Meeting 1993;75:454. Abstract.

5. Bonjour JP, Theintz G, Buchs B, et al. Critical years and stages of puberty for spinal and femoral bone mass accumulation during adolescence. J Clin Endocrinol Metab 1991;73:555–563.

6. Cann CE, Martin MC, Genant HK, Jaffe RB. Decreased spinal mineral content in amenorrheic women. JAMA 1984;251:626–629.

7. Cann CE, Martin MC, Jaffe RB. Duration of amenorrhea affects rate of bone loss in women runners: implications for therapy. Med Sci Sports Exerc 1985;17:214.

8. Cedar MI, Lu JKH, Meldrum DR, Judd HL. Treatment of endometriosis with a long-acting gonadotropin-releasing hormone agonist plus medroxy-progesterone acetate. Obstet Gynecol 1990;75:641–645.

9. Clark N, Nelson M, Evans W. Nutrition education for elite female runners. Phys Sportsmed 1988;16(2):124–136.

10. Davies MC, Hall ML, Jacobs HS. Bone mineral loss in young women with amenorrhea. Br Med J 1990; 301:790–793.

11. de Aloysio D, Mauloni M, Roncuzzi A, et al. Effects of an oral contraceptive combination containing 0.150 mg desogestrel plus 0.020 mg ethinyl estra-diol on healthy premenopausal women. Arch Gynecol Obstet 1993;253:15–19.

12. DeCree C, Lewin R, Ostyn M. Suitability of cyproterone acetate in the treatment of osteoporosis associated with athletic amenorrhea. Int J Sports Med 1988;9:187–192.

13. Dhuper S, Warren MP, Brooks-Gunn J, Fox RP. Effects of hormonal status on bone density in adolescent girls. J Clin Endocrinol Metab 1990;71:1083–1088.

14. Drinkwater BL, Bruemner B, Chesnut CH III. Menstrual history as a deter-minant of current bone density in young athletes. JAMA 1990;263:545–548.

15. Drinkwater BL, Nilson K, Chesnut CH III, et al. Bone mineral content of amenorrheic and eumenorrheic athletes. N Engl J Med 1984;311:277–281.

16. Drinkwater BL, Nilson K, Ott S, Chesnut CH III. Bone mineral density

after resumption of menses in amenorrheic athletes. JAMA 1986;256:380–382.

17. Emans SJ, Grace E, Hoffer FA, et al. Estrogen deficiency in adolescents and young adults: impact on bone mineral content and effects of estrogen replacement therapy. Obstet Gynecol 1990;76:585–592.

18. Finkelstein JS, Neer RM, Biller BMK, et al. Osteopenia in men with a history of delayed puberty. N Engl J Med 1992;326:600–604.

19. Frusztajer NT, Dhuper S, Warren MP, et al. Nutrition and the incidence of stress fractures in ballet dancers. Am J Clin Nutr 1990;51:779–783.

20. Gambacciani M, Spinetti A, Taponeco F, et al. Longitudinal evaluation of perimenopausal vertebral bone loss: effects of a low-dose oral contraceptive preparation on bone mineral density and metabolism. Obstet Gynecol 1994;83:392–396.

21. Genant HK, Cann CE, Ettinger B, Gordan GS. Quantitative computed tomography of vertebral spongiosa: a sensitive method for detecting early bone loss after oophorectomy. Ann Intern Med 1982;97:699–705.

22. Gilsanz V, Gibbens DT, Carlson M, et al. Peak trabecular vertebral density: a comparison of adolescent and adult females. Calcif Tissue Int 1988;43:260–262.

23. Gilsanz V, Gibbens DT, Roe TF, et al. Vertebral bone density in children: effect of puberty. Radiology 1988;166:847–850.

24. Gilsanz V, Roe TF, Mora S, et al. Changes in vertebral bone density in black girls and white girls during childhood and puberty. N Engl J Med 1991;325:1597–1600.

25. Glastre C, Braillon P, David L, et al. Measurement of bone mineral content of the lumbar spine by dual energy x-ray absorptiometry in normal children: correlations with growth parameters. J Clin Endocrinol Metab 1990;70:1330–1333.

26. Hammond CB, Maxson WS. Current status of estrogen therapy for menopause. Fertil Steril 1982;37:5–25.

27. Hohtari H, Salminen-Lappalainen K, Laatikainen T. Response of plasma endorphins, corticotropin, cortisol, and luteinizing hormone in the corticotropin-releasing hormone stimulation test in eumenorrheic and amenorrheic athletes. Fertil Steril 1991;55:276–280.

28. Jonnavithula S, Warren MP, Fox RP, Lazaro MI. Bone density is compromised in amenorrheic women despite return of menses: a 2-year study. Obstet Gynecol 1993;81:669–674.

29. Krolner B, Pors Nielsen S. Bone mineral content of the lumbar spine in normal and osteoporotic women: cross-sectional and longitudinal studies. Clin Sci 1982;62:329–336.

30. Laitinen K, Valimaki M, Keto P. Bone mineral density measured by dual-energy x-ray absorptiometry in healthy Finnish women. Calcif Tissue Int 1991;48:224–231.

31. Lindberg JS, Fears WB, Hunt MM, et al. Exercise-induced amenorrhea and bone density. Ann Intern Med 1984;101:647–648.

32. Lindsay R, Nieves J, Golden A, Kelsey J. Bone mass among premenopausal women. Int J Fertil Menop Stud 1993;38:83–87.

33. Lloyd T, Buchanan JR, Bitzer S, et al. The relationship of diet, athletic activity, menstrual status, and bone density among collegiate women. Am J Clin Nutr 1987;46:681–684.

34. Lloyd T, Rollings N, Andon MB, et al. Determinants of bone density in young women. I. Relationships among pubertal development, total body bone mass, and total body bone density in premenarchal females. J Clin Endocrinol Metab 1992;75:383–387.

35. Lloyd SJ, Triantafyllou SJ, Baker ER, et al. Women athletes with menstrual irregularity have increased musculoskeletal injuries. Med Sci Sports Exerc 1986;18(4):681–684.

36. Loucks AB, Mortola JF, Girton L, Yen SSC. Alterations in the hypothalamic-pituitary-ovarian and the hypothalamic-pituitary-adrenal axes in athletic women. J Clin Endocrinol Metab 1989;68:402–411.

37. Marcus R, Cann CE, Madvig P, et al. Menstrual function and bone mass in elite women distance runners. Ann Intern Med 1985;102:158–163.

38. Mazess RB, Barden HS. Bone density in premenopausal women: effects of age, dietary intake, physical activity, smoking, and birth-control pills. Am J Clin Nutr 1991;53:132–142.

39. McCormick DP, Ponder SW, Fawcett HD, Palmer JL. Spinal bone mineral density in 335 normal and obese children and adolescents: evidence for ethnic and sex differences. J Bone Miner Res 1991;6:507–513.

40. Metka M, Holzer G, Heytmanek G, Huber J. Hypergonadotropic hypogonadic amenorrhea (World Health Organization III) and osteoporosis. Fertil Steril 1992;57:37–41.

41. Neely EK, Marcus R, Rosenfeld RG, Bachrach LK. Turner syndrome adolescents receiving growth hormone are not osteopenic. J Clin Endocrinol Metab 1993;76:861–866.

42. Ott SM. Attainment of peak bone mass. J Clin Endocrinol Metab 1990;71:1082A–1082C. Editorial.

43. Picard D, Ste-Marie LG, Coutu D, et al. Premenopausal bone mineral content relates to height, weight, and calcium intake during early adulthood. Bone and Mineral 1988;4:299–309.

44. Ponder SW, McCormick DP, Fawcett HD, et al. Spinal bone mineral density

in children aged 5.00 through 11.99 years. Am J Dis Child 1990;144:1346–1348.

45. Prior JC, Vigna YM, Schechter MT, Burgess AE. Spinal bone loss and ovulatory disturbances. N Engl J Med 1990;323:1221–1227.

46. Recker RR, Davies KM, Hinders SM, et al. Bone gain in young adult women. JAMA 1992;268:2403–2408.

47. Riggs BL, Eastell R. Exercise, hypogonadism, and osteopenia. JAMA 1986;256:392–393.

48. Rigotti NA, Neer RM, Skates SJ, et al. The clinical course of osteoporosis in anorexia nervosa: a longitudinal study of cortical bone mass. JAMA 1991;265:1133–1138.

49. Rigotti NA, Nussbaum SR, Herzog DB, Neer RM. Osteoporosis in women with anorexia nervosa. N Engl J Med 1984;311:1601–1606.

50. Rosenthal DI, Mayo-Smith W, Hayes CW, et al. Age and bone mass in premenopausal women. J Bone Miner Res 1989;4:533–538.

51. Schlechte JA, Sherman B, Martin R. Bone density in amenorrheic women with and without hyperprolactinoma. J Clin Endocrinol Metab 1983;56:1120–1123.

52. Sowers MF, Kshirsagar A, Crutchfield M, Updike S. Body composition, age, and femoral bone mass of young adult women. Ann Epidemiol 1991;1:245–254.

53. Sugimoto AK, Hodsman AB, Nisker JA. Long term gonadotropin-releasing hormone agonist with standard postmenopausal estrogen replacement failed to prevent vertebral bone loss in premenopausal women. Fertil Steril 1993;60:672–674.

54. Surrey ES, Gambone JC, Lu JKH, Judd HL. The effects of combining norethindrone with a gonadotropin-releasing hormone agonist in the treatment of symptomatic endometriosis. Fertil Steril 1990;53:620–626.

55. Villanueva AL, Schlosser C, Hopper B, et al. Increased cortisol production in women runners. J Clin Endocrinol Metab 1986;63:133–136.

56. Warren MP, Brooks-Gunn J, Fox RP, et al. Lack of bone accretion and amenorrhea: evidence for a relative osteopenia in weight bearing bones. J Clin Endocrinol Metab 1991;72:847–853.

57. Warren MP, Brooks-Gunn J, Hamilton LH, et al. Scoliosis and fractures in young ballet dancers: relation to delayed menarche and secondary amenorrhea. N Engl J Med 1986;314:1348–1353.

58. Warren MP, Holderness CC. Estrogen replacement does not affect bone density with one year of replacement (#425). Endocrine Society Annual Meeting 1992. Abstract.

59. Warren MP, Holderness CC, Lesobre V, et al. Hypothalamic amenorrhea and hidden nutritional insults. J Soc Gynecol Invest 1994;1:84–88.
60. Warren MP, Shane E, Lee MJ, et al. Femoral head collapse associated with anorexia nervosa in a twenty-year-old ballet dancer. Clin Orthop 1990;251:171–176.

The Adult Athlete: Performance-Enhancing Drugs

Anabolic Steroids

The use of anabolic steroids among elite athletes as well as high school and college students is becoming increasingly well known. Perry et al (1990) found that of the 6.6% of high school seniors who currently use or have previously used steroids, the majority started at or before the age of 16. Female steroid users are less common than male, with one source estimating that among older teens, 5% of the males and only 1% of the females use steroids.

Anabolic steroids are synthetic derivatives of testosterone produced to maintain the anabolic and not the androgenic effects of testosterone. Steroids are medically used to treat anemias and to counteract catabolism resulting from trauma or surgery. Athletes and nonathletes use anabolic steroids to increase the size and strength of their muscles, as well as for cosmetic reasons such as reducing body fat content. These steroids have no effect on aerobic performance. Drugs used in training or competition are used for perceived anabolic or performance effects (see Table 10.1).

Mechanisms by Which Steroids Work

Anabolic steroids work by inducing anticatabolic effects, anabolic effects, and motivational effects in the athlete. During stress or intense exercise, endogenous levels of cortisol increase. The catabolic effects of cortisol can lead to a negative nitrogen balance and "muscle wasting" characteristic of an overtrained athlete. The most significant of the three effects of anabolic steroids, the anticatabolic effects, involve reversing the effects of cortisol by displacing it from its receptors.

Table 10.1   *Drugs used by ten women in training or competition*

Anabolic steroids

  Oral

    Mesterolone (Proviron)

    Methandrostenolone (Dianabol [discontinued])

    Methenolone acetate (Primobolan)

    Oxandrolone (Anavar)

    Stanozolol (Winstrol)

  Injectable

    Boldenone undecylenate (Equipoise [veterinary])

    Methandrostenolone ("injectable Dianabol")

    Methenolone enanthate (Primobolan)

    Nandrolone decanoate (Deca-Durabolin)

    Stanozolol (Winston-V [veterinary])

    Stenbolone acetate (Anatrofin)

    Testosterone cypionate

    Mixture of testosterone esters (Sustanon 250)

Growth Hormone

    Somatropin (human growth hormone)

    "Rhesus growth hormone" (a black-market drug of unknown composition)

Analgesic/anti-inflammatory agents

    Acetaminophen and codeine (Tylenol with codeine)

    Aspirin

    Benoxaprofen (Oraflex)

    Naproxen (Naprosyn)

    Oxycodone hydrochloride and aspirin (Percodan)

    Phenylbutazone (Butazolidin)

    Pirozicam (Feldene)

Others

    Epinephrine (adrenalin)

    Ben-Gay (lanolin, menthol, methyl salicylate)

    Caffeine pills

    Calcium

Table 10.1 *Continued*

Choline and inositol

Dimethyl sulfoxide

Electrolyte solution, intravenous

Furosemide (Lasix)

Levodopa

Lidocaine (Xylocaine)

Potassium

Suntan pills

Thyroglobulin

Vitamins

Reproduced by permission from Strauss RH, Liggett MT, Lanese RR. Anabolic steroid use and perceived effects in ten weight-trained women athletes. JAMA 1985;253:2871–2873, p. 2872. Copyright 1985, American Medical Association.

The anabolic mechanisms by which steroids increase size and strength include inducing protein synthesis in muscle cells and stimulating the release of growth hormone, which also has anabolic effects. The motivational effects of steroids are also significant: Athletes who think they are taking steroids but in fact are on placebos show significant strength increases. Athletes have also been shown to become more aggressive on steroids and thus can engage in more rigorous training sessions.

The effects of anabolic steroids are not sustained when discontinued; the increases in muscle size and strength disappear. In males, this is a result of a prolonged suppression of the gonad and severely depleted levels of endogenous testosterone, and in females it results from the loss of exogenous testosterone. In addition, the athlete experiences decreases in motivational influences and aggressive behavior and therefore cannot maintain the intense level of training. To avoid muscle loss, many athletes chronically abuse steroids. Commonly used steroids are listed in Table 10.2, and the perceived changes in a study of 10 female athletes in Table 10.3.

Method and Dosage of Steroid Use

Anabolic steroids can be taken orally or parenterally, and many athletes use a technique called "stacking" in which they take very high doses of a

Table 10.2 *Anabolic steroids reported by heaviest user*
(ten-week cycle)

Drug	Dose	Duration of Use (Weeks)
Oral		
Stanozolol (Winstrol)	12 mg/day	10
Oxandrolone (Anavar)	10 mg/day	10
Mesterolone (Proviron)	50 mg/day	10
Injectable		
Stanozolol (Winstrol-V [veterinary])	50 mg/2 days	last 6
Methenolone acetate (Primobolan)	30 mg/2 days	last 4

Reproduced by permission from Strauss RH, Liggett MT, Lanese RR. Anabolic steroid use and perceived effects in ten weight-trained women athletes. JAMA 1985;253:2871–2873, p. 2872. Copyright 1985, American Medical Association.

combination of 5 or 6 oral and injectable forms simultaneously. This method can induce 10 to 100 times the androgen level of the replacement dosage, and many athletes believe that effects are greater with this method than with a single steroid at the recommended dosage. Many steroid users also believe that each anabolic steroid induces a slightly different effect, and therefore that combinations of steroids will maximize results. A study of 10 female athletes using steroids found that the steroids were taken in a cyclical manner, with the mean cycle length 9.2 (+/−2.2) weeks (typically it is between 4 and 12 weeks), during which a combination of 3.1 (+/−1.7) types of anabolic steroids were used. These women had about 3 menstrual cycles per year, and 4 of the 10 women used lower doses of steroids between cycles. Many studies on toxicity and effectiveness of steroids do not apply to the high dosage level of the multiple ergonic acids that many athletes use. The effects of the orally active and parenterally active compounds are similar, though orally active compounds have been associated with more adverse effects, especially on the liver.

Side Effects of Steroids

Anabolic steroids induce many adverse side effects, including alterations in both the male and female reproductive systems, increased cardiovascular risks, and adverse hepatic, immunologic, endocrinologic, metabolic,

Table 10.3 *Perceived side effects of anabolic steroids in ten women*

Effect	No. Reporting Effect	Perceived as		
		Desirable	Undesirable	Not Significant
Lower voice	10	—	7	3
Facial Hair				
Increased	9	—	8	1
No change	1	—	—	—
Clitoris				
Enlarged	8	2	2	4
No change	2	—	—	—
Libido				
Increased	6	5	1	—
Decreased	1	—	1	—
No change	3	—	—	—
Breast size				
Decreased	5	1	—	4
No change	5	—	—	—
Menstruation				
Diminished or				
stopped	7	3	2	2
Regular	1	—	—	—
Hysterectomized	2	—	—	—
Aggressiveness				
Increased	8	6	2	—
No change	2	—	—	—
Acne				
Increased	6	—	6	—
No change	4	—	—	—
Body Hair				
Increased	5	—	5	—
No change	5	—	—	—
Scalp Hair				
Increased loss	2	—	1	1

Table 10.3 *Continued*

Effect	No. Reporting Effect	Perceived as		
		Desirable	*Undesirable*	*Not Significant*
No change	8	—	—	—
Appetite				
Increased	8	2	5	1
No change	2	—	—	—
Body fat				
Decreased	8	8	—	—
No change	2	—	—	—

Reproduced by permission from Strauss RH, Liggett MT, Lanese RR. Anabolic steroid use and perceived effects in ten weight-trained women athletes. JAMA 1985;253:2871–2873, p. 2872. Copyright 1985, American Medical Association.

and psychological effects. The effects of anabolic steroids are listed in Table 10.4. In males, the steroids mimic endogenous androgens and inhibit the pituitary hypothalamic stimulation of the gonadal producing testosterone, resulting in decreased serum testosterone levels. The testicles consequently atrophy, spermatogenesis diminishes, and transient infertility results. Gynecomastia, possibly a permanent side effect, can develop as the result of the steroid being aromatized to estradiol in the peripheral tissues. Other male reproductive side effects include acne, altered libido, and advancement of male pattern baldness.

The side effects of anabolic steroids in women have been less documented; they include hirsutism, increased muscularity, deepening of the voice, male pattern baldness, hypertrophy of the clitoris, acne, menstrual disorders, and increased aggressiveness. Hirsutism, deepening of the voice, coarsening of the skin, and male pattern baldness may be permanent. Some female steroid users have reported increased libido and a decrease in breast size, although it is unclear whether these are perceived or actual effects.

The orally active anabolic steroids appear to cause adverse effects on the liver, whereas the injectable forms do not. Athletes who use oral steroids may show elevated liver function tests, although it is unclear

Table 10.4 *Effects of anabolic steroids*

Positive effects
  Treatment of catabolic states
  Transient increase in muscular size and strength
    Trauma
    Surgery
Adverse effects
  Cardiovascular
    Increase in cardiac risk factors
      Hypertension
      Altered lipoprotein fractions
      Increase in LDL/HDL ratio
    Reported strokes/myocardial infarctions
  Hepatic effects associated with oral compounds
    Elevated liver enzymes
    Peliosis hepatis (greater than 6 months' use)
    Liver tumors
      Benign
      Malignant (greater than 24 months' use)
  Reproductive system effects
    In males
      Decreased testosterone production
        Abnormal spermatogenesis
        Transient infertility
        Testicular atrophy
    In females
      Altered menstruation
  Endocrine effects
    Decreased thyroid function
  Immunologic effects
    Decreased immunoglobulins IgM/IgA/IgG
  Musculoskeletal effects
    Premature closure of bony growth centers
    Tendon degeneration

Table 10.4 *Continued*

Increased risk of tendon tears

Cosmetic

  In males

    Gynecomastia

    Testicular atrophy

    Acne

    Acceleration of male pattern baldness

  In females

    Clitoral enlargement

    Acne

    Increased facial/body hair

    Coarsening of the skin

    Male pattern balding

    Deepened voice

Psychological

  Risk of habituation

  Severe mood swings

  Aggressive tendencies

  Psychotic episodes

  Depression

  Reports of suicide

Legislation

  Classified as Schedule III controlled substance

Reproduced by permission from Haupt HA. Anabolic steroids and growth hormone. Am J Sports Med 1993;21:468–474, p. 471.

whether this can result from weight lifting alone. Long-term steroid use may cause peliosis hepatis, a condition in which the liver degenerates, and continuous use for more than 24 months may be linked to the development of benign and malignant tumors. Most side effects are transient and reversible upon cessation of steroids.

Increased cardiac risk factors associated with anabolic steroids include significant increases in low-density lipoprotein (LDL), significant decreases in high-density lipoprotein (HDL), and decreases in glucose tolerance and hypertension. Immunologic and endocrine effects include reversible decreases in the immunoglobins IgA, IgG, and IgM; T_3; T_4; thyroid-stimulating hormone (TSH); and thyroxine-binding globulin (TBG). Although these effects are reversible, it is unclear whether an increase in short-term cardiac risk factors may compromise long-term cardiac health, or whether a short-term suppression in immunoglobulins may allow for increased susceptibility to infection.

Steroid users who have not reached their maximum height may experience diminished development as a result of the steroids' possible effect on growth-plate formation with fusion of the epiphysis. The result—shorter height and limbs—is not reversible.

Psychiatric effects are less frequently associated with steroid use, although this may reflect a lack of knowledge about who is taking steroids, since athletes may be reluctant to reveal their steroid use to their physicians. Furthermore, as previously stated, dosages used in research investigations do not represent those actually used by athletes. However, a study of 39 male and 2 female steroid users conducted by Pope and Katz (1988) found that 9 subjects (22%) exhibited a full affective syndrome (including manic and depressive syndromes) and 5 (12%) exhibited psychotic symptoms during a period of steroid use. In comparison, only 2 (4.9%) displayed full affective syndrome while not exposed to steroids. Increased and uncontrolled violence has also been documented with steroid users.

Malarkey et al (1991) conducted a study of 9 female weight lifters using androgens and 7 female weight lifters in their follicular phase who were not using androgens, and found that 7 of the 9 females using androgens had menstrual irregularities. Another central finding of this study was that the mean serum testosterone levels of 7 of the 9 steroid users were 30 times those of the control group or the normal female population, and several had levels higher than normal males. These subjects had the above described symptoms of hyperandrogenism, including enlarged muscles, hirsutism, clitoromegaly, and menstrual irregularities. The androgen users had serum estradiol levels similar to the levels of the controls during the midfollicular phase, suppressed FSH levels, and normal LH levels. Although the values of total cholesterol, LDL cholesterol, and triglyceride did not differ between the two groups, the HDL cholesterol levels were significantly lower in the androgen users. Sex hormone–binding globulin (SHBG), a protein produced in the liver that binds 60% of circulating testosterone, was also lower in women taking androgens.

Steroid Dependence and Withdrawal Symptoms

Dependence on steroids involves both psychological and physiologic factors. Development of an altered body image that is dependent on maintained steroid usage leads to chronic abuse of steroids. This obsession with an altered body image (similar to that seen in anorexia) usually involves complex psychological and emotional issues that need to be approached and treated.

Cessation of steroids can cause a withdrawal syndrome that involves chemically and psychologically based depression. Psychologically, the steroid user loses the sense of power, security, or desirability derived from the steroid-induced physical size and strength, as well as the consequent responses these physical changes may have incited in peers. In addition the athlete experiences a loss of interest in exercise and a decrease in aggression, which consequently diminishes the potential intensity level achieved during exercise. Physically, the athlete experiences a loss of steroid euphoria, and in men, the decrease in testosterone levels causes a loss of sexual interest. To avoid these withdrawal symptoms, the athlete often engages in chronic steroid use, which could lead to unforeseen medical consequences.

With the value society places on physical shape and size, the use of steroids as a shortcut to this end raises complex ethical and health-related issues. In the United States, steroids are not illegal when prescribed by a physician, unless the user is a competing athlete. Still, some athletes who use steroids are permitted to compete. Canada applies a 4-year sanction against athletes who use steroids, and Denmark will imprison for up to 2 years athletes using steroids not medically sanctioned. As of 1990, anabolic steroids are considered a controlled substance that could cause dependence.

Growth Hormone

GH, a peptide hormone produced by somatotroph cells, is the most abundant active protein of the anterior pituitary. It is secreted in a pulsatile manner and affects the growth of almost every organ and tissue in the body except the brain and the eyes. Stimuli that affect the release of GH include sleep (the largest burst of secretion occurs just after the onset of deep sleep), stress, exercise, emotional excitement, and exogenous administration of protein, various drugs, or amino acids. Normal human growth depends on the presence of GH during development. Pituitary dwarfism, a condition that results from low levels or absence of growth hormone, is the only condition legally warranting the exogenous administration of GH. Excessive secretion of endogenous GH causes gigantism in prepubertal subjects and acromegaly in postpubertal subjects.

GH levels vary according to age, sex, fitness, and body composition, with decreased levels in the elderly and obese. GH has hormonal and metabolic influences, and women and adolescents have higher basal levels than adult men. Women show fluctuations in GH levels during various menstrual cycle phases, and women taking estrogens have higher GH levels. Thus it appears that GH release is influenced by estrogen levels, and this is supported by the fact that GH response to release stimuli decreases in menopausal women. GH release does not appear to be influenced by testosterone.

GH release can be increased by psychological and physical stresses, with exercise and hypoglycemia being stimuli for its release. Twenty minutes of exercise at 75% to 90% of maximal oxygen uptake (VO_2max) incites a GH increase equal to that induced by insulin hypoglycemia. GH response is affected by exercise type, intensity, and duration, with intermittent exercise producing higher levels than continuous exercise. GH response to exercise also depends on the individual's sex (with women showing a greater response), level of fitness, and body composition. Obese individuals have a lower GH response to exercise as well as to other exogenous stimuli such as L-dopa.

Growth Hormone and the Athlete

The use of GH as an ergonic acid is less pervasive among athletes than that of anabolic steroids, but athletes do use human GH because they believe that it enhances size and strength and, depending on the age of the user, height. This has not been substantiated by scientific studies, and anecdotal reports vary, with some athletes claiming increases in lean body weight and muscle mass. Animal experiments have shown that GH administration causes an increase in muscle growth but not strength. Although GH use is curtailed by its cost and the requirement of administration with needles, many athletes are drawn to GH because it will bypass current drug detection tests.

Biosynthetic forms of GH, such as somatrem and somatropin, are now available through the use of recombinant DNA technology. Somatrem contains an extra methionine group that causes 30% of children to produce antibodies in response to treatment. Previously GH was obtained from the pituitary glands of human cadavers. This led to a few cases of GH users who developed Creutzfeldt-Jacob disease from cadaver pituitary glands infected with this virus. "Rhesus growth hormone," a black-market substance that has an unknown composition and that may not even contain GH, is cheaper than the costly human growth hormone.

Rather than injecting GH directly, many athletes take amino acid supplements to stimulate their endogenous growth hormone production. It has been shown that arginine, lysine, ornithine, and tryptophan taken alone or in combination can promote endogenous GH release. Release of GH has also been increased by vasopressin, L-dopa, propranolol, and clonidine.

Mechanism of Exogenous Growth Hormone Effects

In studies on several species, GH has caused nitrogen retention and protein accumulation and had a general anabolic effect. GH accelerates amino acid transport into tissues and synthesis into protein. It seems that protein synthesis increases as a result of both the effects of GH and the work of the muscles; the result is an increase in the size of the muscle as compared to muscles untreated with GH. GH decreases cellular glucose uptake, causing an effect opposite to that of insulin, which favors the use of sugar and promotes its conversion to fat. GH conversely triggers the mobilization of lipids from adipose tissue, causing lipids, rather than muscle glycogen, to be used as an energy bank. These effects suggest that GH may cause an increase in strength in an athlete, although the ergonic effects of GH in the athlete are as yet uninvestigated.

In patients with diabetes mellitus, GH causes a diabetogenic effect, but in the nondiabetic patient GH does not significantly change plasma glucose and insulin concentrations. The metabolic effects of GH mimic those of a starved state, with increased intolerance to carbohydrates (hunger diabetes), mobilization of fat, inhibited lipogenesis, and ketosis. Similarly, fasting causes an increase in GH secretion, and thus the use of fat as fuel is diverted from the use of tissue.

Side Effects of Growth Hormone

Excess GH causes acromegaly in the adult, a syndrome characterized by enlargement of the skull and jaw with protruding cheekbones, jaw, and forehead. Hands become wide with thick, oblong fingers, and growth of facial subcutaneous tissue causes features to become coarse. Linear growth of patients with acromegaly does not increase because epiphyseal closure has occurred by the time of adulthood. Muscles appear to increase in size, but in fact they are weak as a result of myopathy. Osteoporosis, diabetes mellitus, hypertension, atherosclerotic heart disease, cardio-myopathy, congestive heart failure, and neuropathy are other complications of acromegaly. Many men with acromegaly may develop impotence, and most women exhibit menstrual dysfunction. Most acromegalics eventually die of cardiac failure, 50% by the age of 50 and 89% by the age of 60. Prepubertal patients with gigantism similarly manifest weak muscles, osteoporosis, and high rate of mortality from cardiac failure. Long-term studies have not been done, but athletes who use GH will be susceptible to the above described symptoms. These problems are difficult to study because GH use is restricted and illegal in this setting. The effects of short-term usage of GH are unknown. The commonly known effects of GH are listed in Table 10.5.

The possession or distribution of GH for unauthorized or nonmedical purposes is punishable by up to 5 years in prison.

Human Chorionic Gonadotropin

The hormone hCG, which is produced by the human placenta and excreted into the urine, stimulates the production of gonadal steroid hormones. If given to females after ovulation it stimulates the corpus luteum to produce progesterone and maintain the placenta; if injected into males it stimulates the Leydig cells to produce testosterone. This is thought to have an indirect anabolic effect by virtue of the increased testosterone levels. hCG is found endogenously in men only in the unusual case of the development of a teratomatous tumor with chorionic elements. The struc-

Table 10.5   *Effects of growth hormone*

Positive effects

   In skeletally immature

      Treatment for pituitary dwarfism

      Increase in height

   In skeletally mature

      Potential increase in muscular size and strength

      Increased use of lipid metabolism as energy source

Adverse effects

   Acromegalic syndrome

      Increased size of facial bones

      Thickened hands and fingers

      Osteoporosis

      Long-term cardiac failure

      Diabetes

      Impotence and amenorrhea

Legislation

   Federal offense to distribute

Reproduced by permission from Haupt HA. Anabolic steroids and growth hormone. Am J Sports Med 1993;21:468–474, p. 472.

ture and mechanism of hCG resembles that of LH, and it is administered to treat infertility in both men and women with gonadotropic deficiency. In women, hCG induces ovulation by simulating a LH surge. hCG is administered by intramuscular injection.

Although hCG has been used to treat obesity, there is no evidence that it affects appetite or lipid mobilization.

Adverse effects of hCG include depression, mood changes, headache, fatigue, restlessness, edema, gynecomastia, precocious puberty, and occasionally production of antibodies to hCG.

Bibliography

1.   Adlercreutz H, Harkonen M, Kuoppasalmi K, et al. Effect of training on plasma anabolic and catabolic steroid hormones and their response during physical exercise. Int J Sports Med 1986;7:27–28.

2. Alen M, Hakkinen K, Komi PV. Changes in neuromuscular performance and muscle fiber characteristics of elite power athletes self-administering androgenic and anabolic steroids. Acta Physiol Scand 1984;122:535–544.

3. Alen M, Rahkila P, Reinila M, Vihko R. Androgenic-anabolic steroid effects on serum thyroid, pituitary and steroid hormones in athletes. Am J Sports Med 1987;15:357–361.

4. American College of Sports Medicine Position Stand. The use of anabolic-androgenic steroids in sports. Med Sci Sports Exerc 1987;19:534–539.

5. Anabolic-androgenic steroids. In: Handbook of experimental pharmacology. Berlin: Springer-Verlag, 1976.

6. Ariel G, Saville W. Anabolic steroids: the physiological effects of placebos. Med Sci Sports 1972;4:124–126.

7. Barr SI. Relationship of eating attitudes to anthropometric variables and dietary intakes of female collegiate swimmers. J Am Diet Assoc 1991;91:976–977.

8. Barron JL, Noakes TD, Levy W, et al. Hypothalamic dysfunction in over-trained athletes. J Clin Endocrinol Metab 1985;60:803–806.

9. Biosynthetic growth hormone. Med Lett Drugs Ther 1985;27:101–104. Editorial.

10. Bonen A, Keizer HA. Athletic menstrual cycle irregularity: endocrine response to exercise and training. Phys Sportsmed 1984;12:78–93.

11. Brower KJ, Blow FC, Beresford TP, Fuelling C. Anabolic-androgenic steroid dependence. J Clin Psychiatry 1989;50:31–33.

12. Brower KJ, Eliopulos GA, Blow FC, et al. Evidence for physical and psychological dependence on anabolic androgenic steroids in eight weight lifters. Am J Psychiatry 1990;147:510–512.

13. Clenbuterol: a new anabolic drug. In: DiPasquale MG, ed. Drugs in sports. vol. 1. Hamilton, Ontario: Decker Periodicals, February 1992:8–10.

14. Cohen JC, Hickman R. Insulin resistance and diminished glucose tolerance in powerlifters ingesting anabolic steroids. J Clin Endocrinol Metab 1987;64:960–963.

15. Conacher GN, Workman DG. Violent crime possibly associated with anabolic steroid use. Am J Psychiatry 1989;146:679.

16. Frankle MA, Cicero GJ, Payne J. Use of androgenic anabolic steroids by athletes. JAMA 1984;252:482.

17. Goodman LS, Gilman A. The pharmacologic basis of therapeutics. 5th ed. New York: Macmillan, 1975.

18. Gribbin HR, Matts SG. Mode of action and use of anabolic steroids. Br J Clin Pract 1976;30:3–9.

19. Haupt HA. Drugs in athletics. Clin Sports Med 1989;8:561–582.

20. Haupt HA. Anabolic steroids and growth hormone. Am J Sports Med 1993;21:468–474.

21. Haupt HA, Rovere GD. Anabolic steroids: a review of the literature. Am J Sports Med 1984;12:469–484.

22. Hays LR, Littleton S, Stillner V. Anabolic steroid dependence. Am J Psychiatry 1990;147:122.

23. Holma PK. Effects of an anabolic steroid (metandienone) on spermatogenesis. Contraception 1977;15:151–162.

24. Houssay AB. Effects of anabolic-androgenic steroids on the skin, including hair and sebaceous glands. In: Kochakian CD, ed. Anabolic-androgenic steroids. New York: Springer-Verlag, 1976:155–190.

25. Hurley BF, Seals DR, Hagberg JM, et al. High-density-lipoprotein cholesterol in bodybuilders v powerlifters: negative effects of androgen use. JAMA 1984;252:507–513.

26. Kashkin KB, Kleber HD. Hooked on hormones? an anabolic steroid addiction hypothesis. JAMA 1989;262:3166–3170.

27. Katzung BG, ed. Basic and clinical pharmacology. 4th ed. Norwalk, Connecticut: Appelton and Lange, 1989:460.

28. Kearns WM. Methyl testosterone administered orally to patients with marked testicular deficiency. J Clin Endocrinol 1941;1:126–130.

29. Kopera H. The history of anabolic steroids and a review of clinical experience with anabolic steroids. Acta Endocrinol Suppl (Copenh) 1985;271:11–18.

30. Kraemer WJ. Endocrine responses to resistance exercise. Med Sci Sports Exerc 1988;20:S152–S157.

31. Kruskemper HL. Anabolic steroids. New York: Academic Press, 1968.

32. Kuret JA, Murad F. Adenohypophyseal hormones and related substances. In: Gilman AG, Rall TW, Nies AS, Taylor P, eds. The pharmacological basis of therapeutics. 8th ed. New York: Pergamon, 1990:1334–1343.

33. Lamb DR. Anabolic steroids in athletics: how well do they work and how dangerous are they? Am J Sports Med 1984;12:31–38.

34. Lemon PWR, Chaney MM. Physiologic effects of amino-acid supplementation. In: Garret WEJ, Malone TR, eds. Muscle development: nutritional alternatives to anabolic steroids, report of the Ross symposium. Columbus: Ross Laboratories, 1988:62–67.

35. Lindberg JS, Fears WB, Hunt MM, et al. Exercise-induced amenorrhea and bone density. Ann Intern Med 1984;101:647–648.

36. Macintyre JG. Growth hormone and athletes. Sports Med 1987;4:129–142.

37. Malarkey WB, Strauss RH, Leizman DJ, et al. Endocrine effects in female weight lifters who self-administer testosterone and anabolic steroids. Am J Obstet Gynecol 1991;165:1385–1390.

38. Martinez JA, Buttery PJ, Pearson JT. The mode of action of anabolic agents: the effect of testosterone on muscle protein metabolism in the female rat. Br J Nutr 1984;52:515–521.

39. Masuda A, Shibasaki T, Hotta M, et al. Insulin-induced hypoglycemia, L-dopa and arginine stimulate GH secretion through different mechanisms in man. Regul Pept 1990;31:53–64.

40. Moffatt R, Wallace M, Sady S. Effects of anabolic steroids on lipoprotein profiles of female weight lifters. Physician Sports Med 1990;18:106–110.

41. Morris DD, Garcia MC. Effects of phenylbutazone and anabolic steroids on adrenal and thyroid gland function tests in healthy horses. Am J Vet Res 1985;46:359–364.

42. Newman S. Despite warnings, lure of steroids too strong for some young Canadians. Can Med Assoc J 1994;151:844–846.

43. Perry PJ, Anderson KH, Yates WR. Illicit anabolic steroid use in athletes: a case series analysis. Am J Sports Med 1990;18:422–428.

44. Pope HG, Katz DL. Affective and psychotic symptoms associated with anabolic steroid use. Am J Psychiatry 1988;145:487–490.

45. Prior JC, Vigna YM, Schechter MT, Burgess AE. Spinal bone loss and ovulatory disturbances. N Engl J Med 1990;323:1221–1227.

46. Problems with growth hormone. Med Lett Drugs Ther 1985;27:57–58. Editorial.

47. Raynaud J, Capderou A, Martineaud JP, et al. Intersubject viability in growth hormone time course during different types of work. J Appl Physiol 1983;55:1682–1687.

48. Reynolds JEF, ed. Martindale: the extra pharmacopoeia. 13th ed. London: Pharmaceutical Press, 1993:949–951.

49. Robbins SL. Pathologic basis of disease. Philadelphia: WB Saunders, 1974.

50. Rodriguez DOL, Valeron MC, Carrillo DA, et al. Evaluation of growth hormone stimulation tests using clonidine, glucagon, propranolol, hypoglycemia, arginine and L-dopa in 267 children of short stature. Rev Clin Esp 1984;173:113–116.

51. Ryan JB, McBride JT. Sports medicine. JAMA 1992;268:411–412.

52. Schedules of controlled substances; anabolic steroids. Federal Register February 13, 1991;56. Rules and Regulations.

53. Senate Bill S.3266-65 Sec. 1904. Amendment to the Food, Drug and Cosmetic Act. Sec. 303 (21 USU §333).

54. Strauss RH, Liggett MT, Lanese RR. Anabolic steroid use and perceived effects in ten weight-trained women athletes. JAMA 1985;253:2871–2873.

55. Sutton J, Lazarus L. Growth hormone in exercise: comparison of physiological and pharmacological stimuli. J Appl Physiol 1976;41:523–527.

56. Use and effects of growth hormone. In: DiPasquale MG, ed. Drugs in sports. vol. 1. Hamilton, Ontario: Decker Periodicals, February 1992:5.

57. Wilson J. Androgen abuse by athletes. Endocrinol Rev 1988;9:181–199.

58. Wilson JD, Griffin JE. The use and misuse of androgens. Metabolism 1980;29:1278–1295.

59. Wright JE. Anabolic steroids and athletes. Exerc Sport Sci Rev 1980;8:149–202.

60. Yesalis CE, Streit AL, Vicary JR, et al. Anabolic steroid use: indications of habituation among adolescents. J Drug Educ 1989;19:103–116.

61. Zekauskas S, Boggs MB, Wilson DP. Human GH and Creutzfeldt-Jakob disease. J Okla State Med Assoc 1990;83:446–448.

CHAPTER 11

The Adult Athlete: Gynecologic Problems and Performance

The Effects of Menses on Athletic Performance

Given the existence of numerous cycle-dependent physical changes, including premenstrual fluid retention, menstrual cramps, and breast tenderness, correlations between cycle phase and athletic performance would seem likely. Wilson et al (1991) found that approximately 50% of female college athletes felt that premenstrual symptoms and dysmenorrhea compromised their athletic ability. However, a study of 12 female recreational weight lifters and 15 female college swimmers conducted by Quadagno et al (1991) indicated that cycle phase did not affect strength or speed in these two groups.

Luteal phase has been associated with lower levels of plasma epinephrine and blood lactate and increased time before exhaustion. Acute exercise has been associated with slight increases in estrogen and progesterone levels, which is a response presumably mediated by decreased clearance through the liver.

Bonen et al (1983) found that cycle phase generally does not effect exercise-induced metabolic changes in subjects. In this study, 19 normally menstruating subjects, divided into a 24-hour fasted group, a glucose-loaded group, and a control group, were studied to investigate substrate and hormonal responses to exercise during the follicular and luteal phases of the cycle and under different nutritional conditions. Independent of menstrual phase, it was found that nutritional status affected exercise-induced responses in glucose, lactate, free fatty acids, insulin, and growth hormone levels. However, within each group, many of the endocrine and substrate responses to exercise were similar in both cycle phases, with the following exceptions. The glucose-rich subjects had a lower free fatty acid response to exercise during the luteal phase. The fasted subjects had elevated insulin and growth hormone responses during the luteal phase, a reduction in LH, and no exercise-induced progesterone increase in the luteal phase. The control group, which had normal nutritional levels, did not differ in substrate or endocrine responses to exercise during each cycle phase, except for a rise in the progesterone response during the luteal phase. This may be related to a reduction in hepatic clearance of steroids during exercise.

Brooks-Gunn et al (1986) investigated performance times of 6 post-menarcheal swimmers for 12 weeks. They found that the fastest times for the 100-yard freestyle and 100-yard best event occurred during menses, and the slowest times during the premenstrual phase. Possible explanations may be effects from premenstrual water retention and subsequent menstrual water reduction. These authors also summarized previous studies that show conflicting data (see Table 11.1).

Menstrual cycle effects on performance probably relate to the amount of perceived distress; no definite conclusions can be drawn from this data. However, severe dysmenorrhea or premenopausal problems would understandably affect performance.

Oral Contraceptives and Athletic Performance

Female athletes are frequently prescribed oral contraceptives (OCs) for therapeutic reasons ranging from contraception to the attenuation of dysmenorrhea. Exercising women commonly express concern about how OCs will affect their sports performance. Since estrogens and progestins can have an impact on a variety of metabolic processes, it is certainly possible that OCs influence athletic performance. However, very little useful, generalizable data addressing this issue are available, and the little available data are inconclusive. The variable dosages of estrogen and progestin in the OCs that are used in research make data interpretation difficult, and differences in the fitness levels of study subjects further complicate analysis. In an early study in which physical education students were given OCs, 46% of subjects observed no difference in performance, and 8% reported a performance improvement. However, as was

Table 11.1 *Athletes exhibiting cycle phase effects (self-reported) in early studies*

Author (Year)	Sample	Cycle Phase Effects: Menstrual and Premenstrual			
		No Cycle Phase Effect (%)	Cycle Phase Performance Decrement (%)	Cycle Phase Performance Enhancement (%)
Erdelyi (1962)	557 athletes (no specific information provided)	42–48	31 (menstrual phase)	13–15 (menstrual phase)
Ingman (1952)	104 Finnish athletes	43	38 (menstrual phase)*	19 (menstrual phase)
Kral and Markalous (1937)	No. of athletes unspecified	63	8 (menstrual phase)	29 (menstrual phase)
Rougier and Linquette (1962)	1435 athletes:	Not specified		
	553 engaged in regular intensive exercise		59 (premenstrual phase, increase in symptoms)	
	309 exercised for 2–4 hrs		11 (premenstrual phase, no increase in symptoms)	
	573 did not exercise			
Zaharieva (1965)	66 athletes in Olympic Games in Tokyo, 1964	37	17 (menstrual phase)	28 (menstrual phase)†

* Of these athletes, 24% did not ordinarily compete during menses because of pain and/or fatigue. This group may account for a large percentage of those reporting poor athletic performances during menstruation.
† Showed a variation in performance, direction not specified.
From Brooks-Gunn J, Garguilo JM, Warren MP. The effect of cycle phase on the adolescent swimmers. Phys Sports Med 1986;14:182–192, p. 184. Reproduced by permission from McGraw-Hill, Inc.

the case in much of the early research relating OCs to performance, data in this study were based on retrospective interviews, a technique known to introduce considerable error. Furthermore, subjects were given preparations with higher dosages of estrogens and progestins than are generally prescribed today.

Researchers have suggested that OC use is associated with a decrease in VO_2max. Dagett et al (1983) observed 7 active women both before and after OC use and found a significant decrease in VO_2max during OC use. When muscle biopsies were performed on women after exogenous steroid use, no significant change was found in muscle lactate or glycogen after exercise, but there was a significant reduction in mitochondrial citrate. However, other researchers have found that OCs have no significant effect on aerobic capacity, and still others report that women on OCs demonstrate a significant increase in oxygen consumption for a standardized workload. Again, none of these studies was carried out using the low-dose triphasic or monophasic formulations that are currently used. A more recent prospective investigation involving a lower-dose OC reported a small but statistically significant reduction in aerobic capacity after 6 months on OCs. This effect was found to be reversed when the hormone administration was discontinued.

Effects of OCs on respiration have also been suggested. The luteal phase has been associated with lower levels of plasma adrenaline and blood lactate and a longer time to exhaustion. Montes et al (1983) found that OCs induced ventilatory changes similar to those occurring during the luteal phase, including increases in tidal volume and expired minute ventilation. Subsequent studies, however, have found no respiratory changes in women taking OCs (LeBrun et al, unpublished data, submitted, 1994). This recent prospective study also showed no significant differences in heart rate between women taking OCs and women in the placebo control group.

The impact of OCs on metabolism, particularly substrate metabolism, remains controversial. Some studies have reported that women taking OCs have lower glucose levels both at rest and during exercise. Others have observed a decrease in carbohydrate metabolism, secondary to a decrease in insulin receptor concentration caused by progestin. Other investigators have found an enhanced GH response during exercise, although this has been disputed.

Finally, it has been hypothesized that OCs have an impact on two other aspects of performance: coordination and strength. In a prospective study of female soccer players, Moller-Nielsen and Hammar (1988) found that women using OCs had a lower rate of traumatic injuries than those who were not on the pill. The authors attribute this to the fact that OCs lead to an amelioration of premenstrual syndrome and dysmenorrhea, which might reduce the risk of injury by affecting coordination. It has been suggested that increases in muscle strength could result from the androgenic component of OCs, based on data from anabolic steroid research. This has never been demonstrated conclusively, though, and is unlikely given the small androgenic component in current OC formulations.

Because of the wide variety of OC preparations currently being used and the relatively small number of studies that have been performed using newer, low-dose formulations, no conclusions can be drawn regarding the effect of currently used OCs on different aspects of athletic performance. It appears that for most women, OCs have no significant effect on athletic performance, but further prospective double-blind studies are needed, particularly using OCs with newer progestins (desogestrel, gestodene, and norgestimate). Future studies should attempt to assess fitness level so that researchers can control for this potentially confounding factor.

Bibliography

Menstrual Cycle and Performance

1. Bonen A, Haynes FJ, Watson-Wright W, Sopper MM, Pierce GN, Low MP, Graham TE. Effects of menstrual cycle on metabolic responses to exercise. J Appl Physiol: Respiratory, Environmental & Exercise Physiology 1983;55(5):1506–1513.
2. Brooks-Gunn J, Gargiulo JM, Warren MP. The effects of cycle phase on the adolescent swimmers. Phys and Sports Med 1986;14:182–192.
3. Jurkowski JE, Jones NL, Toews CJ, Sutton JR. Effects of menstrual cycle on blood lactate, O_2 delivery, and performance during exercise. J Appl Physiol 1981;51:1493–1499.
4. Jurkowski JE, Sutton JR, Klare P. Effect of the menstrual cycle on the plasma catecholamine response to exercise in normal females. Can J Appl Sport Sci 1978;3:194.

5. Keizer HA, Rogol AD. Physical exercise and menstrual cycle alterations: what are the mechanisms? Sports Med 1990;10:218–235.

6. Loucks AB, Mortola JF, Girton L, Yen SSC. Alterations in the hypothalamic-pituitary-ovarian and the hypothalamic-pituitary-adrenal axes in athletic women. J Clin Endocrinol Metab 1989;68:402–411.

7. Quadagno D, Faquin L, Lim G, et al. The menstrual cycle: does it affect athletic performance? Physician Sports Med 1991;19:121–124.

8. Wilson CA, Abdenour TE, Keye WR. Menstrual disorders among intercollegiate athletes and nonathletes: perceived impact on performance. Athletic Training J Natl Athletic Trainers Assoc 1991;26:170–177.

Oral Contraceptives and Performance

1. Bale P, Davies J. Effect of menstruation and contraceptive pill on the performance of physical education students. Sports Med 1983;17:46–50.

2. Bemben DA, Boileau RA, Bahr JM, et al. Effects of oral contraceptives on hormonal and metabolic responses during exercise. Med Sci Sports Exerc 1992;24:434–441.

3. Daggett A, Davies B, Boobis L. Physiological and biochemical responses to exercise following oral contraceptive use. Med Sci Sports Exerc 1983; 15:174.

4. Erdelyi GJ. Gynecological survey of female athletes. J Sports Med 1962; 2(September):174–179.

5. Huisveld IA, Hospers JEH, Bernick MJ, et al. The effect of oral contraceptives and exercise on hemostatic and fibrinolytic mechanisms in trained women. Int J Sports Med 1983;4:97–103.

6. Ingman O. Menstruation in Finnish top-class sports women. International symposium of the medicine and physiology of sports and athletes, Helsinki, Finnish Association of Sportsmedicine, 1952:96–98.

7. Kral J, Markalous E. The influence of menstruation on sport performance, in Proceeding of the 2nd International Congress on Sports Medicine, New York City, Thieme-Stratton, 1937.

8. Lebrun CM. The effect of the phase of the menstrual cycle and the birth control pill on athletic performance. Clin Sports Med 1994;13:419–441.

9. McNeill AW, Mozingo E. Changes in the metabolic cost of standardized work associated with the use of an oral contraceptive. J Sports Med Phys Fitness 1981;21:238–244.

10. Moller-Nielsen J, Hammar M. Women's soccer injuries in relation to the menstrual cycle and oral contraceptive use. Med Sci Sports Exerc 1988; 21:126–129.

11. Montes A, Lally D, Hale RW. The effects of oral contraceptives on respiration. Fertil Steril 1983;39:515–519.
12. Notelovitz M, Zauner C, McKenzie L, et al. The effect of low-dose contraceptives on cardiorespiratory function, coagulation, and lipids in exercising young women: a preliminary report. Am J Obstet Gynecol 1987;156:591–598.
13. Prior JC, Vigna YM. Gonadal steroids in athletic women: contraception, complications, and performance. Sports Med 1985;2:287–295.
14. Rougier G, Linquette Y. Menstruation and physical exercise. Presse Med 1962;70(October):1921–1923.
15. Zaharieva E. Survey of sportswomen at the Tokyo Olympics. J Sports Med 1965;5(December):215–219.

The Pregnant Athlete

Until fairly recently, most physicians advised their pregnant patients to avoid exercising, regardless of their previous exercise habits, their medical conditions, or their obstetrical courses. Little was known about the effects of exercise upon pregnancy and of pregnancy upon exercise, and most physicians assumed that avoidance of exercise presented the safest advice. Many pregnant women exercised anyway, either disregarding the advice of their physicians or strategically failing to ask for such advice. The lack of adverse outcomes in most such pregnancies, the increased numbers of women who were exercising regularly, and the emphasis on women's health care led a handful of concerned investigators to seek information about exercise and pregnancy, thereby providing answers to many of these questions.

At one time it seemed reasonable to advise all pregnant women to rest as much as possible and to avoid strenuous exertion. That advice is no longer acceptable. Many women find it necessary to be physically active for financial, social, or personal reasons, and many others choose an active lifestyle because they enjoy it and believe it is beneficial in many ways. Recent studies have provided much more important information about the effects of exercise upon pregnancy and pregnancy outcome and about the effects of pregnancy upon exercise and training.

Physiologic Changes

Many physiologic alterations occur during the course of a normal pregnancy, including cardiovascular, hemodynamic, pulmonary, metabolic, and endocrine changes and alterations in weight, weight distribution,

113

body composition, size, and nutritional requirements. Regular physical exercise and training also lead to alterations in these systems and factors. The combined changes observed from pregnancy and training often enhance those produced by either one alone.

Cardiovascular Alterations

Pregnancy   One of the most striking alterations that occurs during pregnancy is the very large increase in blood volume, averaging 45% to 50% by term in 20% to 100% of women, depending on size and parity. This is accompanied by a great increase in cardiac output, reaching a maximum increment of more than 50% above nonpregnant levels by late pregnancy. Cardiac output is the product of stroke volume and heart rate, both of which increase during pregnancy. Stroke volume rises by 8 weeks of gestation and continues to increase to its maximal level during the second trimester. Heart rate response to exercise also varies widely among individuals and varies with position and gestational age. Left ventricular mass increases because of increased wall thickness. Accompanying the increases in cardiac output and blood volume are decreases in systemic vascular resistance and diastolic blood pressure. Although venous pressure in the upper body remains fairly constant, venous pressure in the lower extremities increases significantly with advancing gestational age as a result of partial obstruction of the inferior vena cava and the common iliac veins by the uterus and presenting fetal part. The increased cardiac output that occurs throughout pregnancy is accompanied by large increases in blood flow to the uterus, placenta, kidneys, and skin.

Exercise and Training   Acute exercise leads to an increase in cardiac output, proportional to the intensity of the exercise. The major increment in cardiac output supplies the exercising skeletal muscle, and a smaller increment supplies the heart. Most of the other organs receive the same or a reduced portion of cardiac output during exercise.

The cardiac output response during exercise is greater during pregnancy than in the nonpregnant state. The pregnancy-induced rise in cardiac output at low exercise intensities is related to increases in both heart rate and stroke volume. At higher exercise intensities, however, increases in stroke volume account for more of the gain in cardiac output than do increases in heart rate.

Fitness

Exercise   Specific types of endurance training are known to increase cardiovascular fitness, as assessed by measurements of VO_2max. VO_2max represents our best measurement of cardiovascular fitness, reflecting the maximal amount of oxygen that can be taken in, delivered, and utilized. Among nonpregnant athletes, cross-country skiers and distance runners have the highest recorded values of VO_2max, as a result of their endurance training.

Pregnancy and Training   Anecdotal observation suggests that for many athletes who trained throughout pregnancy, the pregnancy resulted in a training effect, leading to improved athletic performance after the pregnancy. Recent studies have confirmed that this does, in fact, occur. Postpregnancy measurements of VO_2max in athletes who trained throughout pregnancy exceed similar prepregnancy measurements.

Hemodynamic Alterations

Pregnancy   Red blood cell mass increases throughout pregnancy. However, plasma volume increases earlier in pregnancy and at a faster rate than the rise in red blood cell mass, causing a dilutional anemia that worsens until the second trimester and then remains at a plateau. Plasma volume expansion correlates with infant birth weight and favorable outcome, and failure of plasma volume expansion during pregnancy has been associated with lower birth weight and fetal growth retardation. The isoosmotic plasma volume expansion that occurs during pregnancy is accompanied by an increase in total extracellular volume, not just plasma volume.

Exercise and Training   Chronic endurance training also leads to an increased blood volume, partly due to an increase in intravascular plasma protein content. Red blood cell volume also expands with chronic training, but this increase is less than that occurring in plasma volume. As a result, chronic exercise also causes a dilutional anemia.

The combined effects of pregnancy and endurance training produce hemodynamic changes that are greater than those seen with either pregnancy or training alone. Thus, during the second and third trimesters, pregnant exercisers demonstrate greater blood volume, plasma volume, and red blood cell volume compared to sedentary pregnant women.

Pulmonary Alterations

Pregnancy   During normal pregnancy, tidal volume increases, total lung capacity decreases, functional residual capacity decreases, residual volume decreases, expiratory reserve volume decreases, alveolar ventilation increases, and inspiratory capacity increases. In addition, respiratory rate increases slightly, tidal volume increases appreciably, and oxygen consumption increases moderately. Respiratory minute volume increases, causing a decrease in alveolar CO_2.

Exercise and Training   Exercise ventilation during pregnancy increases more than oxygen uptake, possible because of a direct effect of progesterone and an increased sensitivity to carbon dioxide.

Endocrine and Metabolic Alterations

Pregnancy   Pregnancy, an anabolic state, is accompanied by increased plasma levels of insulin, estrogen, progesterone, prolactin, and human placental lactogen. Insulin leads to increased synthesis of glycogen, protein, fatty acids, and lipids, resulting in lower plasma levels of glucose, amino acids, and free fatty acids. Fat accumulation and increased protein synthesis begin early in pregnancy, partly in response to higher circulating levels of insulin and to insulin resistance.

Fat accumulation ceases during the second half of pregnancy, when cortisol, GH, and insulin concentrations continue to rise, and fetal energy requirements rise even more dramatically. Although fasting levels of glucose, amino acids, free fatty acids, and ketones remain fairly constant throughout pregnancy, prolonged fasting (longer than 6 hours) leads to a decrease in blood glucose and amino acids and to an increase in free fatty acids and ketones.

Exercise and Training   During exercise, pregnant women experience a decrease in blood concentrations of glucose and insulin and a rise in free fatty acids. The catecholamine response to exercise that occurs in the nonpregnant state is blunted during pregnancy, thereby impairing the glycogenolysis and glucose production that normally correct hypoglycemia in the nonpregnant state. Significant hypoglycemia can occur following exercise in the second and third trimesters of pregnancy, and this may be of concern for some exercising women.

Thermoregulation

Pregnancy   Maternal temperature is normally about 0.5°C higher than follicular phase temperatures, as a result of the thermogenic effect of progesterone. Fetal temperature is normally about 0.5°C higher than maternal temperature, due primarily to the higher fetal and placental metabolic rates that result from growth and development. This fetal-maternal temperature gradient ensures that fetal heat is always transferred to the mother and represents the only mechanism by which the fetus can dissipate heat.

Exercise   The fetal-maternal temperature gradient of 0.5°C observed at rest is initially reduced during exercise and is eventually reversed during prolonged maternal exercise, as maternal temperature rises. This reversal of the fetal-maternal temperature gradient leads to a transfer of heat from mother to fetus. Animal studies have demonstrated that the fetal temperature quickly exceeds the maternal temperature as a result of maternal heat dissipation, and fetal temperature may remain elevated for more than one hour and probably for several hours (see Figure 12.1). The fetal-maternal temperature gradient may easily exceed the normal resting fetal-maternal temperature gradient of 0.5°C and may reach levels of 1.0°C. Thus, the fetal temperature can remain significantly elevated long after the maternal temperature has returned to normal.

Alteration in Weight

Pregnancy   Maternal weight gain during pregnancy includes the fetus, the placenta, amniotic fluid, the uterus, the breasts, intravascular fluid, and adipose tissue. Insufficient maternal weight gain may compromise fetal growth and development; excessive maternal weight gain promotes accumulation of maternal adipose tissue.

Training   Endurance exercise training promotes less weight gain than occurs in sedentary women, and cessation of training promotes weight gain. Such weight gain exceeds that gained by either sedentary women or those who continue exercising regularly.

Pregnant exercisers show similar effects: Those who continue exercising throughout pregnancy gain less weight than sedentary pregnant women,

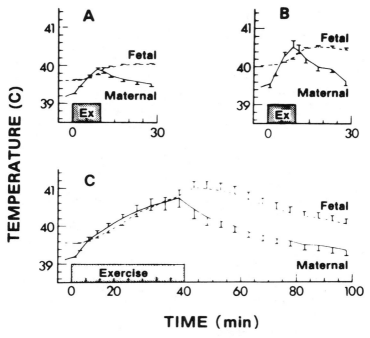

Figure 12.1 *Maternal and fetal temperature changes in response to three different exercise regimens. Values are means ± SE, (n = 6). A: 10-min exercise at 70% maximal oxygen consumption (VO₂max), B: 10-min exercise at 100% VO₂max, C: 40-min exercise at 70% VO₂max. (Reproduced by permission from Lotgering FK, Gilbert RD, Longo LD. Excercise responses in pregnant sheep: blood gases, temperature, and fetal cardiovascular system. J Appl Physiol 1983;55:842–850.)*

who gain less weight than pregnant exercisers who cease exercising by the twenty-eighth week of gestation. The offspring of those who continue exercising throughout pregnancy have lower birthweights than those of sedentary pregnant women, whose offspring have lower birthweights than the offspring of pregnant exercisers who cease exercising by the twenty-eighth week of gestation.

Joint Alteration

Pregnancy   Several investigators have demonstrated progressive development of maternal peripheral joint laxity throughout pregnancy. The cause and consequences of these joint changes remain to be shown.

Table 12.1 *Nutritional needs for pregnancy and exercise*

	Increased Requirement for	
	Pregnancy	Exercise
Calories	↑	↑
Protein	↑	–
Fat	–	–
Carbohydrate	↑	↑
Vitamins	↑	↑/–
Minerals	↑	–
Water	–	↑

Alterations in Nutritional Requirements

Pregnancy   Pregnancy leads to increased requirements for calories, protein, carbohydrate, most vitamins, and several minerals.

Training   Exercise leads to increased requirements for calories, carbohydrates, a few vitamins, and water. Among vitamins, only thiamine, niacin, riboflavin, and pantothenic acid are dependent upon energy expenditure. The combination of pregnancy and exercise, therefore, increases a woman's needs for calories, protein, carbohydrate, most vitamins, several minerals, and water (see Table 12.1).

Safety of Exercise

Concerns about the safety of exercise during pregnancy have focused on several major issues: blood flow, temperature, nutrient availability, and trauma. Since scientific research has demonstrated that exercise and training are beneficial in general, it has been assumed that exercise is beneficial to pregnant women too. Questions about safety have always addressed the fetus, about whom less information was available and less could be gathered within the ethical guidelines required by sound judgment and morality.

Blood Flow and Distribution

As discussed previously, exercise is accompanied by increased blood distribution to the heart and exercising skeletal muscle and reduced blood distribution to splanchnic and other intra-abdominal organs. Exercise intensity correlates directly with the increased blood flow to exercising skeletal muscle and correlates indirectly with reduced uterine blood flow in animal studies (see Figure 12.2). It is not known at what intensity humans can exercise without experiencing a diversion of blood from the uterus. Some animal data suggest that when exercise reduces uterine blood flow, it shifts preferentially toward the placenta and away from the myometrium. This would certainly be a favorable situation if it occurs in humans. However, the studies needed to confirm or disprove this probably cannot be performed in humans, so the answers may never be found.

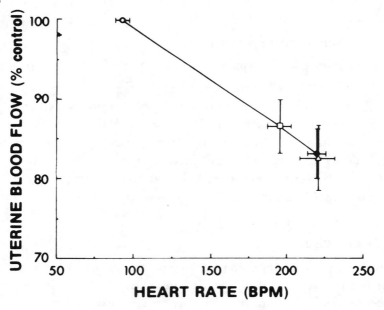

Figure 12.2   *Uterine blood flow response to 3 different exercise regimens in pregnant sheep (n = 8). Values are means ± SE. A: 10-min exercise at 70% maximal oxygen consumption (VO$_{2max}$), B: 10-min exercise at 100% VO$_{2max}$, C: 40-min exercise at 70% VO$_{2max}$. (Reproduced by permision from Lotgering FK, Gilbert RD, Longo LD. Excercise responses in pregnant sheep: oxygen consumption, uterine blood flow, and blood volume. J Appl Physiol 1983;55:834–841.)*

Although no data have been published to confirm or disprove the existence of a critical exercise intensity for safety, or variability among individuals in such a critical exercise intensity level, it is likely that both exist. A critical threshold of exercise—above which uterine or placental blood flow is reduced and below which uterine and placental blood flow remain adequate for normal fetal growth, development, and well-being—probably exists but likely varies greatly among individuals. This threshold may even vary in the same individual at different stages of pregnancy or at different levels of fitness.

Fetal Heart Rate   Among the most reliable parameters used to assess and monitor fetal well-being is fetal heart rate. Several investigators have monitored fetal heart rate before, during, and after exercise. Findings indicate a brisk fetal heart rate elevation following moderate maternal exercise.

Among the older studies addressing fetal heart rate during maternal exercise, one that has received much attention and wide citation was published by Morris et al (1956). The investigators studied effective blood flow during normal and pre-eclamptic pregnancies and found a decrease in effective uterine blood flow during moderately intense supine cycling. Since the supine position itself can decrease uterine blood flow as a result of decreased cardiac output from decreased venous return due to inferior vena caval compression, it is unclear whether the observed decrease in uterine blood flow resulted from the exercise, the supine position, or both. Unfortunately, most citations of this publication referred only to the observed decrease in uterine blood flow during exercise without reference to the supine position of the exercising subjects. The conclusion of authors and critics of this study was that exercise is dangerous for the fetus, and many years passed before this idea was challenged. However, it is certainly prudent for pregnant exercisers to avoid any exercises performed in the supine position.

During the past decade several researchers have studied the effects of maternal exercise upon fetal heart rate. Some investigators have reported fetal bradycardia during maternal exercise, when measured by Doppler ultrasound, but these measurements have been shown to reflect motion artifact during maternal exercise. Thus two-dimensional M-Mode echocardiography is believed to assess the fetal heart rate during maternal exercise with greater accuracy than does Doppler ultrasound.

Carpenter et al (1988) subjected 45 pregnant women to a total of 79 maximal exercise tests and 85 submaximal tests (see Figure 12.3). The authors reported that three episodes of fetal bradycardia occurred in association with submaximal exertion: one before exercise, one during a vasovagal hypotensive episode during exercise, and one following exercise. Fifteen episodes of fetal bradycardia occurred following maximal exertion; in most cases, onset occurred within two minutes after cessation of maximal exertion and termination occurred within a few minutes after onset of bradycardia. However, three of these episodes of bradycardia lasted longer than 9 minutes (see Figure 12.4). These important findings suggest that it is prudent to advise pregnant women to avoid maximal exertion when they exercise.

The 15 episodes of bradycardia that occurred in association with exercise took place following cessation of maximal exertion, but none occurred during the actual maximal exertion. Perhaps this interesting observation can be attributed to the hemodynamic changes associated with acute exercise during pregnancy. Immediately following cessation of acute exertion, heart rate, stroke volume, and cardiac output all decrease

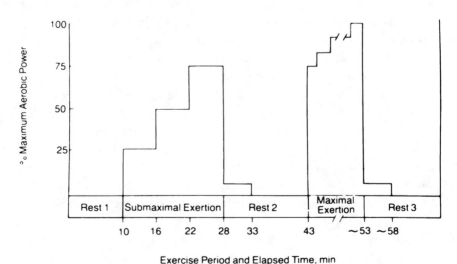

Exercise Period and Elapsed Time, min

Figure 12.3 *Exercise protocol: duration of rest and exercise periods and associated percentage of maximal aerobic power. (Reproduced by permission from Carpenter MW, Sady SP, Hoegsberg b. et al. Fetal heart rate response to maternal exertion. JAMA 1988;259:3006–3009.)*

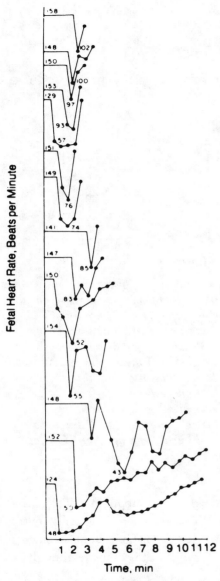

Figure 12.4   *Fetal heart rate following maximal exertion during 14 episodes of fetal bradycardia. Fetal heart rates were averaged over 10 cardiac cycles every 30 s during postexercise period. One tape was lost. Predeceleration baseline fetal heart rate and nadir fetal heart rate are noted for each deceleration. Zero time equals time of cessation of maximal exertion. (Reproduced with permission from Carpenter MW, Sady SP, Hoegsberg b. et al. Fetal heart rate response to maternal exertion. JAMA 1988;259:3006–3009.)*

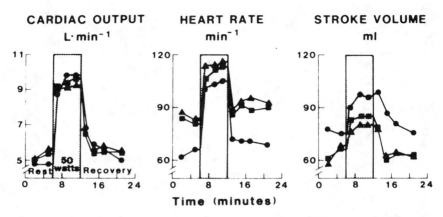

Figure 12.5 *Cardiac output and its components, heart rate, and stroke volume are shown at rest, during 50W upright bicycle exercise, and during recovery at 34 and 38 weeks' gestation, and 3 months postpartum. Measurements of cardiac output, heart rate, and stroke volume were not different at 34 and 38 weeks' gestation; these results were averaged to provide a single late-gestation measurement. Although cardiac output was not affected by late gestation during this exercise protocol, the heart rate and stroke volume responses differed in late gestation compared to the postpartum period. (Reproduced by permission from Morton MJ, Paul MS, Campos FR, et al. Exercise dynamics in late gestation: effects of physical training. Am J Obstet Gynecol 1985;152:91–97.)*

sharply (see Figure 12.5). It may be that a combination of decreased uterine perfusion during strenuous exercise and decreased cardiac output immediately following strenuous exertion predisposes some women to acute, transient placental insufficiency, which leads to the fetal bradycardia noted by the investigators.

Pregnancy Outcome

Pregnancy outcome can be assessed by perinatal morbidity and mortality, by birth weight, and by neonatal growth and development. Although studies have demonstrated higher litter mortality in rats trained during pregnancy regardless of prepregnancy training, no similar effects have been shown in humans. Differences have been observed among animal species in their responses to exercise during pregnancy, and it remains unclear whether conclusions about humans can be drawn from any of the animal species that have been studied. To date, scientific studies have demonstrated no adverse effects from exercise in the periconceptual period and throughout pregnancy upon the incidence of failure to conceive, spontaneous abortion, congenital abnormalities, abnormal placentation, premature rupture of the membranes, or preterm labor.

Temperature

Significant exercise stress in animals is often associated with maternal hyperthermia and respiratory alkalosis, both of which have been shown to result in decreased uterine perfusion. Fetal hyperthermia in animals can lead to cardiovascular collapse and death.

Animal studies have confirmed the detrimental effects of maternal hyperthermia, especially prior to closure of the neural groove, and pregnant animals exposed to hyperthermia prior to this embryologic event have a higher risk of neural tube defects. Although the relevance of these animal data to humans remained unclear and has been questioned for a long time, it appears quite convincing that these effects can occur in humans too. The neural groove closes after approximately 23 to 28 days of gestation in humans. Maternal hyperthermia in early pregnancy carries a potential risk for neural tube defects and, in later pregnancy, for intrauterine growth retardation.

To date, no cases of maternal hyperthermia have been reported in association with exercise, nor have any cases of congenital anomalies. Although no human cases of abnormal development or intrauterine growth retardation have been linked to exercise-induced hyperthermia, neural tube defects have been observed in the offspring of women who were exposed to high temperatures in early pregnancy during sauna use or febrile illnesses. It is still unknown whether animal data can be extrapolated to humans, but the potential risks of teratogenic effects in early pregnancy and intrauterine growth retardation in later pregnancy must be taken seriously.

Nutrient Availability

As mentioned previously, inadequate provision of caloric needs may lead to intrauterine growth retardation, and excessive provision of calories may lead to accumulation of maternal adipose tissue. Pregnant exercisers must be very attentive to food and fluid intake because the usual signals of hunger, appetite, and thirst may be modified by pregnancy hormones. That is, food and nutrient intake may be limited by nausea in early pregnancy and by reduced stomach capacity in late pregnancy. As a result, the pregnant exerciser must remain vigilant of her caloric intake and expenditure in order to provide adequate needs for both the pregnancy and the exercise.

Fluid intake should be increased to offset fluid lost in perspiration. Pregnant exercisers should be particularly attentive to fluid intake because dehydration augments the thermogenic effects of exercise and may lead to maternal hyperthermia, especially in hot weather.

Trauma

Certain sports and activities present potential risks for fetal trauma or premature placental separation as a result of sudden impact. However, in early pregnancy, the fetus is sufficiently protected by the bones and muscles of the maternal pelvis, and, in later pregnancy, the fetus is generally well protected by amniotic fluid. Thus, the risks imposed by trauma remain theoretical to date.

Recommended Guidelines

Types of Exercise

Endurance Exercise   Pregnancy is hard work, and most women should be advised to become physically fit before becoming pregnant. However, fitness is a desirable goal for all women during pregnancy, even for those who lacked this foresight, as long as no medical or obstetrical complications exist or arise.

Aerobic exercise is desirable and is necessary to achieve cardiovascular fitness. Safe limits for aerobic exercise have not been determined, and this point should be emphasized to all pregnant exercisers. The amount of aerobic exercise that a pregnant woman should undertake depends upon her previous exercise habits and fitness levels. It is appropriate to counsel all pregnant women about exercise, providing advice about intensity, duration, and frequency, as well as specific activities.

Pregnant women can probably continue any aerobic exercise they were accustomed to performing at the same perceived level of exertion practiced prior to pregnancy. Because pregnancy increases the workload of any woman, even at rest, and because body weight increases throughout pregnancy, exercise during pregnancy represents a much greater workload than in the nonpregnant state. Although an increase in efficiency offsets these increments somewhat, pregnant exercisers at all stages of pregnancy are performing more work than they did in the nonpregnant state. As a result, pace should be slower and should probably be adjusted by perceived exertion.

Heart rate is not a reliable indicator for many women, particularly since it varies widely throughout pregnancy, with position, and among individuals. However, heart rate is a quantifiable measurement, and some exercisers may feel more comfortable with such a tool. In such a case, it is appropriate to tell patients that very intensive exercise during pregnancy (accompanied by heart rates exceeding 150 beats per minute) has been associated with brief fetal bradycardia, although without any observed adverse consequences. It is important to encourage gradual slowing down after cessation of exercise, rather than stopping abruptly. Sudden cessation of exercise leads to a drastic decrease in heart rate, stroke volume, and cardiac output, which may promote transient reductions in uterine blood flow and consequential fetal bradycardia.

Safe duration of aerobic exercise has not been determined. However, it is likely that sessions of 30 minutes or less are unlikely to present dangers from changes in either blood flow or temperature. Little is known about the effects of prolonged exertion or about exertion under environmental extremes of high heat, humidity, or altitude. Until these conditions are shown to be safe, they should be avoided. Longer durations of exercise may increase the risks from prolonged diversion of uterine blood flow and from hyperthermia. It is advisable for every pregnant exerciser to check her rectal temperature once in early pregnancy, immediately after completion of her customary exercise routine. This assessment should probably be repeated at monthly intervals afterward. Rectal temperatures of less than 101°F probably reflect safe workouts. Higher recorded temperatures should lead to modifications in the exercise routine (clothing, pace, intensity, or environment), in order to maintain a lower core temperature.

Safe frequency of aerobic exercise has not been determined either. However, it is likely that exercise frequencies as short as twice daily are safe, as long as fetal growth is adequate. Since fitness can be attained and maintained with less frequent workouts, it is unlikely that many athletes will choose to exercise so often. For those who were accustomed to longer durations of exercise prior to pregnancy, though, and who wish to exercise more frequently in order to compensate for reduced exercise duration, workouts as frequent as twice daily or even more often will probably offer a safe and reasonable solution. For those women exercising to achieve cardiovascular fitness, an exercise frequency of 3 or 4 times a week will probably meet their needs and goals.

Women who were not accustomed to aerobic exercise prior to pregnancy can be encouraged to practice walking, which is also a good choice for those who find it uncomfortable to continue their previous activities. Walking permits comfortable pacing and is well suited to those exercising alone. Activities such as aerobics are often difficult and uncomfortable for many women to continue throughout pregnancy because the group of individuals in any class represent different levels of fitness and perform different workloads at their own varied body weights and gestational ages. For this reason, individual sports offer pregnant women the best opportunity to pace themselves comfortably, using their own comfort levels (and possibly heart rates) to set their own paces.

Aerobic exercise should be avoided by women with any of the following conditions: premature labor, ruptured membranes, multiple gestation, incompetent cervix, cardiac disease, intrauterine growth retardation, or other medical or obstetric complications that make such exercise unwise.

Weight Training   Weight training (resistance training) is probably safe during pregnancy, even for those who never practiced it prior to pregnancy. However, no scientific studies have shown the safety of weight training during pregnancy, and none have proven any benefit from weight training during pregnancy either. Weight training should be avoided by those who have cardiac disease, hypertension, or musculoskeletal injuries. Weight training will strengthen muscles and bones, and stronger muscles will probably facilitate maternal activity throughout later pregnancy, when the combination of added body weight, altered center of gravity, and weak low back muscles often promote musculoskeletal pain. Stronger muscles will also facilitate caring for the neonate and carrying the equipment and supplies necessary to provide such care.

Stretching   Exercises that stretch muscles are safe for all pregnant women, even those who never exercised before. Stretching helps to promote flexibility by preventing the shortening that often occurs as muscles heal following exertion. Stretching exercises are safest when practiced after muscles have been warmed by exercising.

Food and Fluid Intake

Pregnant exercisers must eat enough to provide energy for themselves, the growing fetus, and the exercise. Appetite is not a reliable guide for many pregnant women because it may be increased or decreased by hormonal and physical changes from the pregnancy itself, unrelated to true energy requirements. Women may lose a few pounds during the first trimester because of nausea; in the third trimester, the gravid uterus may compress the stomach, limiting appetite and eating capacity. Pregnant exercisers should monitor their food intake and energy expenditures to be sure that caloric needs are being met.

Both pregnancy and exercise increase requirements for calories and some vitamins and minerals. These added needs can be met by increasing food intake, especially with nutrient-rich whole grains, fruits, vegetables, and dairy products, rather than with low-nutrient or high-fat foods. Although some women can provide all of their vitamin and mineral requirements through dietary sources alone, most will benefit from a prenatal vitamin and mineral supplement to ensure that supplies are adequate. Iron stores are often low and will be improved by iron supplementation for most pregnant women. Dietary calcium is usually inadequate for most women, and calcium supplementation is advisable for most women of all ages.

Pregnant exercisers should try to maintain good hydration, probably by ingesting even more fluids than would be suggested by thirst alone. As mentioned previously, dehydration exacerbates hyperthermia, and thirst is not a good indicator of dehydration. Pregnant exercisers should be advised to drink water before, during, and after exercising. They should monitor urine output carefully, paying special attention to frequency, volume, and concentration of urine.

Weight Gain

Pregnant exercisers should be advised to gain about 25 to 40 lbs by term gestation. In 1990, the Subcommittee on Nutritional Status and Weight

Gain during Pregnancy of the Food and Nutrition Board of the Institute of Medicine recommended that total weight gain during pregnancy should be adjusted on the basis of the mother's prepregnancy body mass index (BMI = weight/height^2), as follows: underweight women (BMI less than 19.8) should gain 28 to 40 lbs; normal weight women (BMI from 19.8 to 26.0) should gain 25 to 35 lbs; overweight women (BMI from 26.0 to 29.1) should gain at least 15 lbs. No distinction was made for exercisers, and it is not known whether different recommendations should be made for those who continue exercising throughout pregnancy or for those who discontinue exercising at some time during pregnancy. Until different advice is available for pregnant exercisers, they should be encouraged to follow these guidelines.

Specific Dangers

Pregnant women should be advised to avoid any sport or activity that may lead to low oxygen availability, hyperthermia, abdominal trauma, or supine hypotension. Thus, the following sports should be avoided during

Table 12.2 *Sports recommended throughout pregnancy*

Walking	Racquetball	Waterskiing
Jogging	Squash	Downhill skiing
Hiking	Paddleball	Cross-country skiing
Aerobic dancing	Handball	Rowing
Other fast dancing	Tennis	Canoeing
Weight training	Badminton	Ice skating
Calisthenics	Swimming	Roller skating
Bicycling	Volleyball	Archery
Baseball	Golf	Yoga
Softball	Bowling	Javelin
Basketball	Frisbee	Discus
Touch football	Sailing	Table tennis

Reproduced by permission from Shangold M, Mirkin G. Pregnancy and afterward. In: Shangold M, Mirkin G. The complete sports medicine book for women, Revised Edition. New York: Fireside 1992, p. 141.

Table 12.3 *ACOG recommendations for exercise in pregnancy and postpartum*

There are no data in humans to indicate that pregnant women should limit exercise intensity and lower target heart rates because of potential adverse effects. For women who do not have any additional risk factors for adverse maternal or perinatal outcome, the following recommendations may be made:

1. During pregnancy, women can continue to exercise and derive health benefits even from mild-to-moderate exercise routines. Regular exercise (at least three times per week) is preferable to intermittent activity.

2. Women should avoid exercise in the supine position after the first trimester. Such a position is associated with decreased cardiac output in most pregnant women; because the remaining cardiac output will be preferentially distributed away from splanchnic beds (including the uterus) during vigorous exercise, such regimens are best avoided during pregnancy. Prolonged periods of motionless standing should also be avoided.

3. Women should be aware of the decreased oxygen available for aerobic exercise during pregnancy. They should be encouraged to modify the intensity of their exercise according to maternal symptoms. Pregnant women should stop exercising when fatigued and not exercise to exhaustion. Weight-bearing exercises may under some circumstances be continued at intensities similar to those prior to pregnancy throughout pregnancy. Non-weight-bearing exercises such as cycling or swimming will minimize the risk of injury and facilitate the continuation of exercise during pregnancy.

4. Morphologic changes in pregnancy should serve as a relative contraindication to types of exercise in which loss of balance could be detrimental to maternal or fetal well-being, especially in the third trimester. Further, any type of exercise involving the potential for even mild abdominal trauma should be avoided.

5. Pregnancy requires an additional 300 kcal/d in order to maintain metabolic homeostasis. Thus, women who exercise during pregnancy should be particularly careful to ensure an adequate diet.

6. Pregnant women who exercise in the first trimester should augment heat dissipation by ensuring adequate hydration, appropriate clothing, and optimal environmental surroundings during exercise.

Table 12.3 *Continued*

7. Many of the physiologic and morphologic changes of pregnancy persist 4–6 weeks postpartum. Thus, prepregnancy exercise routines should be resumed gradually based on a woman's physical capability.

Contraindications to Exercise

The aforementioned recommendations are intended for women who do not have any additional risk factors for adverse maternal or perinatal outcome. A number of medical or obstetric conditions may lead the obstetrician to recommend modifications of these principles. The following conditions should be considered contraindications to exercise during pregnancy.

- Pregnancy-induced hypertension
- Preterm rupture of membranes
- Preterm labor during the prior or current pregnancy or both
- Incompetent cervix/cerclage
- Persistent second- or third-trimester bleeding
- Intrauterine growth retardation

Reproduced by permission from American College of Obstetricians and Gynecologists. Exercise During Pregnancy and the Postpartum Period. ACOG Technical Bulletin 189. Washington, DC: ACOG 1994, pp. 3–4.

pregnancy: competitive track and field (except for javelin and discus), boxing, fencing, hockey, soccer, tackle football, hang gliding, skydiving, scuba diving, springboard diving, mountain climbing, and parachute jumping.

Women who experience pain, bleeding, rupture of membranes, or absence of fetal movement should stop exercising and should not resume exercising until it has been determined that they can do so safely.

Resuming Exercise After Pregnancy

It is probably safe for any woman to resume exercising after delivery when she can do so without any pain. Following a vaginal delivery, this may be as early as the first postpartum day, but most exercisers will prefer to wait at least a few days. Following a cesarean delivery, exercisers may be able to resume light exercise (both aerobic and weight training) as early as the seventh postpartum day; intense aerobic exercise, strenuous weight training, and any water sports should be postponed for at least three weeks following a cesarean birth (see Tables 12.2 and 12.3).

Bibliography

1. Artal R, Platt L, Sperling M, et al. Exercise in pregnancy I. Maternal cardiovascular and metabolic responses in normal pregnancy. Am J Obstet Gynecol 1981;140:123–127.
2. Artal R, Wiswell R, Romem Y, et al. Pulmonary responses to exercise in pregnancy. Am J Obstet Gynecol 1986;154:378–383.
3. Blackburn MW, Calloway DH. Heart rate and energy expenditure of pregnancy and lactating women. Am J Clin Nutr 1985;42:1161–1169.
4. Calguneri M, Bird HA, Wright V. Changes in joint laxity occurring during pregnancy. Anri Rheum Dis 1982;41:126–128.
5. Capeless EL, Clapp JF. Cardiovascular changes in early phase of pregnancy. Am J Obstet Gynecol 1989;161:1449–1453.
6. Carpenter MW, Sady SP, Sady MA, et al. Effect of maternal weight gain during pregnancy on exercise performance. J Appl Physiol 1990;68:1173–1176.
7. Carpenter MW, Sady SP, Hoegsberg B, et al. Fetal heart rate response to maternal exertion. JAMA 1988;259:3006–3009.
8. Chandler KD, Bell AW. Effects of maternal exercise on fetal and maternal respiration and nutrient metabolism in the pregnant ewe. J Dev Physiol 1981;3:161–176.
9. Clapp JF. Cardiac output and uterine blood flow in the pregnant ewe. Am J Obstet Gynecol 1978;130:419–423.
10. Clapp JF. Acute exercise stress in the pregnant ewe. Am J Obstet Gynecol 1980;136:489–494.
11. Clapp JF. Maternal heart rate in pregnancy. Am J Obstet Gynecol 1985;152:659–660.
12. Clapp JF. The effects of maternal exercise on early pregnancy outcome. Am J Obstet Gynecol 1989;161:1453–1457.
13. Clapp JF. The course of labor after endurance exercise during pregnancy. Am J Obstet Gynecol 1990;163:1799–1805.
14. Clapp JF. The changing thermal response to endurance exercise during pregnancy. Am J Obstet Gynecol 1991;165:1684–1689.
15. Clapp JF. A clinical approach to exercise during pregnancy. Clin Sports Med 1994;13:443–458.
16. Clapp JF, Capeless EL. Neonatal morphometrics after endurance exercise during pregnancy. Am J Obstet Gynecol 1990;163:1805–1811.

17. Clapp JF, Capeless E. The VO_2max of recreational athletes before and after pregnancy. Med Sci Sports Exerc 1991;23:1128–1133.

18. Clapp JF, Dickstein S. Endurance exercise and pregnancy outcome. Med Sci Sports Exerc 1984;16:556–562.

19. Clapp JF III, Jackson MR, Rizk K, et al. Regular exercise during pregnancy improves placental growth and functional capacity. Med Sci Sports Exerc 1994;26(suppl):118. Abstract.

20. Clapp JF, Rokey R, Treadway JL, et al. Exercise in pregnancy. Med Sci Sports Exerc 1992;24(suppl):S294–S300.

21. Clapp JF, Wesley M, Sleamaker RH. Thermoregulatory and metabolic responses to jogging prior to and during pregnancy. Med Sci Sports Exerc 1987;19:124–130.

22. Clark SL, Cotton DB, Pivarnik JM, et al. Position change and central hemodynamic profile during normal third-trimester pregnancy and post partum. Am J Obstet Gynecol 1991;164:883–887. Am J Obstet Gynecol 1991;165:241. Erratum.

23. Collings CA, Curet LB, Mullin JP. Maternal and fetal responses to a maternal aerobic exercise program. Am J Obstet Gynecol 1983;145:702–770.

24. Curet LB, Orr JA, Ranking JHG, Ungerer T. Effect of exercise on cardiac output and distribution of uterine blood flow in pregnant ewes. J Appl Physiol 1976;40:725–728.

25. Durnin JV. Energy requirements of pregnancy. Diabetes 1991;40(suppl): 152–156.

26. Erkkola R. The influence of physical training during pregnancy on physical work capacity and circulatory parameters. Scand J Clin Lab Invest 1976;36:747–754.

27. Erkkola R, Rauramo L. Correlation of maternal physical fitness during pregnancy with maternal and fetal pH and lactic acid at delivery. Acta Obstet Gynecol Scand 1976;55:441–446.

28. Gorski J. Exercise during pregnancy: maternal and fetal responses. A brief review. Med Sci Sports Exerc 1985;17:407–416.

29. Hall DC, Kaufmann DA. Effects of aerobic and strength conditioning on pregnancy outcomes. Am J Obstet Gynecol 1987;157:1199–1203.

30. Harvey MAS, McRorie MM, Smith DW. Suggested limits to the use of the hot tub and sauna by pregnant women. Can Med Assoc J 1981;125:50–53.

31. Knuttgen HG, Emerson K. Physiological response to pregnancy at rest and during exercise. J Appl Physiol 1974;36:549–553.

32. Lokey EA, Tran ZV, Wells CL, et al. Effects of physical exercise on pregnancy outcomes: a meta-analytic review. Med Sci Sports Exerc 1991; 23:1234–1239.

33. Lotgering FK, Gilbert RD, Longo LD. Exercise responses in pregnant sheep: oxygen consumption, uterine blood flow, and blood volume. J Appl Physiol 1983;55:834–841.

34. Lotgering FK, Gilbert RD, Longo LD. Exercise responses in pregnant sheep: blood gases, temperature and fetal cardiovascular system. J Appl Physiol 1983;55:842–850.

35. Lotgering FK, Gilbert RD, Longo LD. Maternal and fetal responses to exercise during pregnancy. Physiol Rev 1985;65:1–36.

36. McMurray RG, Hackney AC, Katz VL, et al. Pregnancy induced changes in the maximal physiological responses during swimming. J Appl Physiol 1991;71:1454.

37. McMurray RG, Mottola MF, Wolfe LA, et al. Brief review: recent advances in understanding maternal and fetal responses to exercise. Med Sci Sports Exerc 1993;25:1305–1321.

38. Milunsky A, Ulcickas M, Rothman KJ, et al. Maternal heat exposure and neural tube defects. JAMA 1992;268:882.

39. Morris N, Osborn SB, Wright HP, et al. Effective uterine blood flow during exercise in normal and pre-eclamptic pregnancies. Lancet 1956;2:481–484.

40. Morrow RJ, Knox Ritchie JW, Bull SB. Fetal and maternal hemodynamic responses to exercise in pregnancy assessed by Doppler ultrasonography. Am J Obstet Gynecol 1989;160:138–140.

41. Morton MJ, Paul MS, Campos GR, et al. Exercise dynamics in late gestation: effects of physical training. Am J Obstet Gynecol 1985;152:91–97.

42. Paolone AM, Shangold M, Paul D, et al. Fetal heart rate measurement during maternal exercise. J Appl Physiol 1987;62:848–849.

43. Paolone AM, Shangold M, Paul D, et al. Fetal heart rate measurement during maternal exercise—avoidance of artifact. Med Sci Sports Exerc 1987;19:605–609.

44. Pivarnik JM, Lee W, Clark SL, et al. Cardiac output responses of primigravid women during exercise determined by the direct Fick technique. Obstet Gynecol 1990;75:954–959.

45. Pivarnik JM, Lee W, Miller JF. Physiological and perceptual responses to cycle and treadmill exercise during pregnancy. Med Sci Sports Exerc 1991;23:470–475.

46. Pleet H, Graham JM, Smith DW. Central nervous system and facial defects associated with maternal hyperthermia at four to fourteen weeks gestation. Pediatrics 1981;67:785–789.

47. Pomerance JJ, Gluck L, Lynch VA. Physical fitness in pregnancy: its effect on pregnancy outcome. Am J Obstet Gynecol 1974;119:867–876.

48. Rauramo I, Forss M. Effects of exercise on placental blood flow in pregnancies complicated by hypertension, diabetes or intrahepatic cholestasis. Acta Obstet Gynecol Scand 1988;67:15–20.

49. Robson SC, Hunter S, Boys RJ, et al. Serial study of factors influencing changes in cardiac output during human pregnancy. Am J Physiol 1989;256:H1060–H1065.

50. Sady SP, Carpenter MW, Sady MA, et al. Prediction of VO_2max during cycle exercise in pregnant women. J Appl Physiol 1988;65:657–661.

51. Subcommittee on Nutritional Status and Weight Gain During Pregnancy, Institute of Medicine. Nutrition during pregnancy. Washington, D.C.: National Academy Press, 1990.

52. Ueland K, Novy MJ, Metcalfe J. Cardiorespiratory responses to pregnancy and exercise in normal women and patients with heart disease. Am J Obstet Gynecol 1973;115:4–10.

53. Veille JC, Hohimer AR, Burry K, et al. The effect of exercise on uterine activity in the last eight weeks of pregnancy. Am J Obstet Gynecol 1985;151:727–730.

54. Voitk AJ, Mueller JC, Farlinger DE, et al. Carpal tunnel syndrome in pregnancy. Can Med Assoc J 1983;128:277–281.

55. Wilson NC, Gisolfi CV. Effects of exercising rats during pregnancy. J Appl Physiol 1980;48:34–40.

CHAPTER 13

The Athlete at Menopause

Menopause and Exercise

Many older women were socially programmed to be sedentary adults because sedentary behavior was associated with femininity during their formative years. The tremendous publicity given to the benefits of regular exercise has caught the attention of this group, who now require individualized instruction. A program of regular exercise can prevent or minimize many problems of later life, such as cardiovascular disease, obesity, muscle weakness, osteoporosis, and depression. In providing primary care to these women, it is our responsibility to encourage them to develop and maintain regular exercise programs and convince them that such exercise is necessary.

To understand how exercise and training affect the symptoms and problems of menopausal women, it is useful to review the normal physiologic changes accompanying menopause, as well as causes and related etiologic factors.

Menopause

Definition and Physiology　Menopause, the final cessation of menstruation, occurs when functioning ovarian follicles become depleted and cease production of estradiol. This event occurs at an average age of 52 in the United States. Maximum follicular number is attained at approximately 20 weeks of gestation, at which time the average female fetus has about 6 million ovarian follicles. As a result of follicular atresia and, to a much lesser extent, cyclic ovulation during the reproductive years, the number of follicles diminishes to approximately 10 to 50 thousand by menopause, at which time very few are functioning and none are functioning normally.

Effect of Exercise   Exercise and training have no effect on the age at which menopause occurs. Although some athletes experience primary or secondary amenorrhea, these conditions are very different from menopause and can be distinguished from it by measurement of serum concentrations of FSH. FSH is markedly elevated (greater than 40 mIU/ml) following menopause; FSH is low or normal in exercise-associated amenorrhea.

Perimenopausal Bleeding Patterns   As a woman approaches menopause, she produces less estrogen, and cycles become abnormal prior to total cessation of bleeding. During the 5 to 10 years proceeding menopause and for about 5 years afterward, she is hormonally different from the way she was before and from the way she will be afterward. This "climacteric" is often accompanied by symptoms of estrogen deficiency and fluctuation. During the climacteric years that precede menopause, the menstrual interval (the number of days from the onset of one menstrual period until the onset of the next menstrual period) may be shortened and bleeding may be lighter. The earliest menstrual change a woman experiences as she approaches menopause is usually a luteal phase defect, marked by shortening of the luteal phase and lower progesterone concentrations in that phase. It is common for perimenopausal women to experience shortening of both the follicular phase and the luteal phase, due to abnormal follicular maturation in these aging follicles. Next, cycles usually become anovulatory, as follicular maturation becomes inadequate to trigger ovulation. This pattern leads to chronic unopposed estrogen stimulation of the endometrium, which may progress to endometrial hyperplasia and even adenocarcinoma if it continues long enough, unless it is detected and treated. This progression is more likely to take place in women producing significant amounts of estrogen from adipose tissue rather than from ovarian follicles alone. In women producing reduced amounts of estrogen from aging ovarian follicles, the resultant endometrial stimulation usually leads to lighter menstrual flow and a prolonged menstrual interval. The normal progression toward menopause includes progressively lighter flow and longer intervals. However, shorter intervals may also represent a normal progression, as long as flow is lighter. Heavier bleeding always warrants evaluation by endometrial biopsy, regardless of whether the interval is shorter than 25 days or longer than 35 days. Unless heavier bleeding with a normal interval (25 to 35 days) has an obvious explanation (such as uterine myomata), it too warrants evaluation by endometrial biopsy.

Symptoms and Problems   The major symptoms of menopause are vasomotor symptoms (hot flashes and night sweats) and vaginal dryness. The hormonal cause of vasomotor instability has not been identified; vaginal dryness results from urogenital atrophy due to estrogen deficiency. Other problems that are associated with menopause, such as osteoporosis and cardiovascular disease, produce no symptoms until the disease is very advanced. These occur more frequently in estrogen-deficient women.

Several factors besides menopause also influence conditions such as osteoporosis and cardiovascular disease and make it difficult to isolate etiologies. For example, aging, diet, and lack of exercise influence bone density and cardiovascular health. Estrogen, exercise, and dietary calcium enhance bone density and reduce bone loss. Conversely, estrogen deficiency, lack of exercise, and inadequate dietary calcium accelerate bone loss and reduce bone density. Estrogen, regular aerobic exercise, and a low-fat diet reduce the risk of cardiovascular disease. Conversely, estrogen deficiency, lack of aerobic exercise, and a high-fat diet increase the risk of cardiovascular disease. Thus, it is often difficult to separate aging, menopause, and the cumulative effects of an adverse lifestyle when determining the cause of symptoms and problems experienced by menopausal women.

Depression is another problem common among menopausal women, and many women attribute this problem to menopause. However, many types of depression are not related to menopause or the hormonal changes accompanying it. Women who experience frequent vasomotor symptoms at night and sleep disturbances may develop depression as a result of chronic sleep deprivation, which can also lead to a variety of mood and behavioral changes. These women will probably benefit from estrogen therapy. However, most depressed women require treatment with psycho-tropic medication (serotonin receptor agonists or serotonin uptake inhibitors) rather than with estrogen. Recent data suggest, however, that women on estrogen may respond more positively to antidepressant therapy.

Obesity, too, is common among menopausal women, and many women attribute their weight gain to menopause. However, there is no scientific evidence linking obesity and menopause or the hormonal changes accompanying it. It is much more likely that menopause is a time when a woman notices many body alterations that have occurred gradually without her prior notice. Accumulation of adipose tissue occurs gradually with aging, especially in sedentary women. The weight gain that accompanies the aging process is not affected by menopause or hormone replacement therapy.

Benefits of Exercise

Regular aerobic exercise and weight training can benefit all men and women. Fortunately, menopausal status does not alter the beneficial effects of exercise. Because many of the problems that affect women at and after menopause are favorably influenced by exercise, women in these age groups stand to benefit from such exercise even more than many younger women.

Cardiovascular Disease

The risk of cardiovascular disease rises with increasing age among people of both sexes. Regular aerobic exercise (exercise done continually at a sustained elevated heart rate) can help to reduce this risk. Women reporting higher levels of activity tend to have more favorable cardiovascular risk profiles than less active women, when lipid and carbohydrate profiles are compared. Higher levels of physical activity are associated with lower blood pressure, heart rate, serum cholesterol, LDL cholesterol, triglycerides, BMI, skinfold thickness, fasting insulin, and fasting insulin–glucose ratios as well as with higher HDL cholesterol.

The beneficial effects of aerobic exercise training upon cardiovascular disease risk include not only reduction of metabolic risk factors but also improvement in aerobic cardiorespiratory endurance. Pollock (1978) has

shown that male endurance runners of any age were more fit than sedentary men of the same age. He a' 'o demonstrated that older endurance
runners were more fit than young sedentary men, thereby suggesting that
men can become more fit with increasing age.

Several investigators have shown that cardiorespiratory endurance in
women also improves with aerobic training. In investigating how fitness
can be achieved, Pollock determined that VO_2max was higher following
a program of running, walking, and cycling compared to the pretraining
baseline level. Each of these training programs comprised 30 minutes of
continual exercise in the sport, carried out 3 times each week for 20
weeks. These data suggest that any form of aerobic exercise can improve
cardiovascular fitness.

Pollock also showed that those who exercised for 45 minutes in each
session had greater improvement in fitness than those who exercised
30 minutes in each session; these in turn had greater improvement
in fitness than those who exercised only 15 minutes in each session.
He found, too, that those who exercised 5 times a week had greater
improvement in fitness than those who exercised 3 times a week, who in
turn had greater improvement in fitness than those who exercised only
once a week.

When he assessed the injury rate, Pollock found that those who exercised 45 minutes in each session had a higher injury rate than those
who exercised 15 minutes. He also noted that those who exercised
five times a week had a higher injury rate than those who exercised
three times or once a week. Based on these data, he recommended that
in order to improve cardiovascular fitness without incurring a
significant risk of injury, men should exercise for 30 minutes three times
a week.

Pollock's findings form the basis of all current recommendations
for aerobic exercise programs. Although this landmark study was carried
out in men, similar findings have been demonstrated more recently in
women.

Obesity

One of the unfortunate changes accompanying the aging process for most
people is an increase in body fat, and excessive body fat is a problem for
many older women. Although there is no evidence that this condition is

related to menopause, it is a common belief among many women that their fat accumulation began or increased at this time.

It is commonly believed that the average woman permanently adds some weight with each pregnancy, and several studies have supported this contention. However, other investigations have demonstrated that the increase in BMI experienced by the average woman over time is the same, regardless of whether she has an intervening pregnancy.

The importance of regional fat distribution has been demonstrated by the finding that abdominal fat is a risk factor for cardiovascular disease and diabetes, while femoral fat is not statistically associated with these diseases. Aerobic exercise promotes loss of abdominal fat more readily than fat at other sites and promotes loss of fat more readily in men than in women. The sensitivity of abdominal fat to exercise is beneficial in its reduction of disease. However, the relative resistance of femoral fat stores to exercise may be discouraging to many women, particularly since women tend to deposit fat more easily in this region.

The most common cause of obesity is inactivity. When Pollock assessed body fat in the same group of men described previously, he found that the young endurance runners had less body fat than the sedentary men of the same age. He also noted that the older endurance runners had less body fat than the younger sedentary men, thereby suggesting that men can become thinner with increasing age. Similar findings have been demonstrated in women as well.

Most older women try to control their weight and body fat by caloric restriction, but fat is lost much more effectively by exercising than by dieting. The effectiveness of exercise in promoting loss of fat results from several mechanisms, including energy expenditure, metabolic rate, and altered body composition. It has been shown that in both young and middle-aged male exercisers, the time spent training correlates with body composition, energy requirements, and aerobic capacity. Energy expenditure is directly related to time spent exercising, and body fat is inversely related to time spent exercising. Most importantly, exercise reverses the depressed metabolic rate produced by severe caloric restriction. Resting metabolic rate correlates directly with fat-free mass, thereby suggesting that a muscular woman will have a greater metabolic rate than a fat woman of the same weight. The only way to increase lean body mass is, of course, by exercising.

Muscle Weakness

Another common accompaniment of the aging process is loss of both muscle tissue and muscle strength. Many older women lack sufficient strength to remain functional and independent. The age-related decline in lean body mass correlates with several alterations: a decrease in endogenous GH, a decrease in pituitary responsiveness to growth hormone releasing hormone (GHRH), loss of muscle fibers, neuromuscular alteration, inactivity, and other age-related changes. Although premenopausal women have significantly greater pituitary response to GHRH than do men of the same age, postmenopausal women do not. This observation suggests that postmenopausal estrogen deficiency accelerates the age-related decrease in GH secretion and may also accelerate the loss of muscle tissue that occurs as women age. Older men have demonstrated an increase in both lean body mass and skin thickness and a decrease in adipose tissue in response to treatment with GH, but this has not been investigated in older women. Moreover, the safety of such therapy has not yet been determined.

Several investigations have demonstrated a loss of muscle strength with age, beginning after the third decade of life and amounting to a loss of about 16% or more. This loss is greater in women than in men and correlates with several important metabolic activities, including a decrease in basal metabolic rate.

Resistance exercise is the most effective way to increase and maintain muscle strength. Older women require specific instruction to learn such techniques, particularly since in most cases this type of exercise was never taught to them before. Women can significantly improve their strength by participating in regular weight training programs. A desirable program for achieving and maintaining muscle strength should include several resistance exercises using a number of different muscle groups and should be practiced once or twice each week. Such a program should be initiated under supervision for women lacking previous experience in this technique, but it may be continued safely without supervision once the participant feels comfortable and confident.

Osteopenia and Osteoporosis

Physiologic Changes in Bone Mass and Density Both osteopenia and osteoporosis are serious consequences of the aging process. Lower levels of estrogen following menopause appear to be the most important cause of bone loss, but inactivity is an important determinant too. Bone is active tissue that is constantly undergoing formation and resorption. Exercise is one of the few known means of stimulating new bone formation. Bone mass and density diminish when the rate of formation fails to keep pace with the rate of resorption. Cortical bone constitutes about 80% of the total skeleton but is metabolically less active than trabecular (cancellous) bone. Only about 10% of the cortical bone is remodeled every year. Trabecular bone is found in the axial skeleton, primarily in the vertebral bodies, and lesser concentrations are found in the femoral neck and the distal radius. Approximately 40% of trabecular bone is remodeled every year. As a result of this greater activity of trabecular bone, vertebral osteoporosis occurs more often than hip fractures.

After completion of long bone growth, bone mineral content and bone mass continue to increase until about age 35, at which time maximal cortical bone mass is achieved. It is considered normal for women to lose at least 0.12% of cortical bone annually between the time at which peak bone mass is reached and the time of menopause; during the next 10 to 15 years, the rate of bone loss increases to at least 1% annually; subsequently, the rate of loss slows to approximately 0.18% annually. This physiologic bone loss averages out to a 25% decrease in cortical bone mass over the 30 years from age 50 to age 80 and a 32% decrease in trabecular bone mass over the 50 years from age 30 to age 80. Those women who have achieved a greater peak bone mass will be less likely to experience an osteoporotic fracture than those who have achieved lower peak bone mass. Thus, all women should be encouraged to maximize peak bone mass during the early years of bone accrual, as well as to minimize subsequent bone loss.

Effects of Estrogen and Estrogen Deficiency Estrogen increases intestinal absorption of calcium and decreases bone resorption of calcium. Estrogen deficiency accelerates bone loss and undoubtedly accounts for the increased rate of loss during the first five years after menopause. Women who experience estrogen deficiency prior to menopause lose bone mass as a result and are at markedly increased risk of developing osteoporosis in later years.

Effect of Exercise   Mechanical force stimulates bone formation, but minimum requirements remain unknown. Studies have shown that the same exercises that improve muscle strength are beneficial for improving bone density. Such investigations have demonstrated that postmenopausal women can increase bone density in the distal radius following a 5-month program of light arm exercise practiced 3 times a week. These data suggest that bone density can be increased at any site if adequate stress is provided to that bone or to the muscles attached to it. Other studies have reported a direct correlation between physical fitness and femoral neck bone mineral density in both premenopausal and postmenopausal women, probably because regular physical exercise promotes both fitness and bone density.

Body weight correlates with bone density, and this correlation represents the only beneficial effect of obesity. Those who lose weight by dieting or smoking cigarettes lose this beneficial effect of obesity, while those who lose weight by exercising retain this benefit—the favorable effect of the exercise helps to offset the reduced body weight. Cigarettes adversely affect bone density by other means as well. Thus women should be encouraged to exercise for this reason too.

Vasomotor Symptoms

Physically active postmenopausal women experience fewer and milder vasomotor symptoms than do inactive women of the same age and menopausal status. The explanation for this remains unknown.

Depression and Mood Alteration

Regular exercise leads to improvement in mood, presumably as a result of brain production of mood-elevating chemicals. It is believed that these include norepinephrine, epinephrine, cortisol, serotonin, and β-endorphins. However, serum levels of these chemicals do not correlate with brain concentrations, and it is unknown if exercise alters the blood-brain barrier. Exercise has been prescribed for treatment of depression, and it is likely that many depressed people are treating themselves by exercising.

Risks of Exercise

Cardiovascular Disease

Although regular aerobic exercise decreases the risk of cardiovascular disease, those who have coronary artery disease are at greater risk for myocardial ischemia and infarction during exertion. Thus it is important to identify those with cardiovascular disease and to be sure that their exercise programs are reasonable and supervised.

Musculoskeletal Disease

Those with existing musculoskeletal disease may be at increased risk of injury to specific muscles, bones, or joints and may have to select exercise programs that avoid affected areas. For example, women with osteoarthritis should probably exercise uninvolved joints, and women with osteopenia should avoid subjecting affected bones to excessive force. Those with specific acute injuries should avoid exercising injured muscles and joints.

It remains controversial whether repeated microtrauma during weight-bearing exercises, such as running, predisposes involved joints to osteoarthritis. Osteoarthritis is very common among older women, even though fewer than one-third of women with diagnosed osteoarthritis are symptomatic. Since osteoarthritis of the knee correlates with obesity, it is likely that regular exercise helps to prevent this condition. Once osteoarthritis is established, however, the exercise program should be reassessed to incorporate necessary modifications to avoid pain and joint damage.

Other Diseases

Women with abnormalities in carbohydrate metabolism (such as diabetes mellitus) may require modification of their medication schedules and dosages because exercise increases glucose utilization and insulin sensitivity. Similar adjustments in medication may be needed for other specific diseases for which exercise affects symptoms or metabolism of medication. Enumeration of such conditions extends well beyond the scope of this text.

Women with specific medical diseases should undertake and continue regular exercise programs with the advice of the specialist treating their disease. For each woman, a plan should be devised to enable her to exercise in a way that promotes cardiovascular fitness and muscular strength without incurring pain or risk of injury. Each woman should exercise muscle groups that are not involved by the disease process, and she should strengthen the affected areas within the limits imposed by their conditions.

Gynecologic Issues

Stress Urinary Incontinence

Stress urinary incontinence is involuntary leakage of urine during any "stress" or increase in intra-abdominal pressure. This is a relatively common problem among older women, parous women, exercising women, obese women, and women with chronic coughs. However, urine leakage occurs whenever intravesical pressure exceeds intraurethral pressure. Although stress urinary incontinence is most likely to result in those women who have an anatomic defect in the posterior ureterovesical angle, even women with normal anatomy can experience this annoying leakage when intravesical pressure rises sufficiently. Physical activity raises intra-abdominal pressure whenever the Valsalva maneuver is performed, and this occurs commonly during running, jumping, and weight training.

Alterations in intra-abdominal pressure are not always transmitted equally to both bladder and urethra, and intravesical pressure often exceeds intraurethral pressure as a result. Although stress urinary incontinence occurs more commonly during exercise than during rest, exercise-induced increases in intra-abdominal pressure are transient and do not lead to chronic pressure alterations or anatomic defects.

Pelvic relaxation includes several anatomic defects with loss of support, including cystocele, urethrocele, rectocele, and uterine descensus. These anatomic abnormalities are often related to previous obstetrical trauma and with endogenous joint hypermobility. Such joint laxity may also predispose certain women to joint injury. Women with obvious anatomic defects usually require surgical correction of their problems. Repeated increases in pressure postoperatively may lead to a recurrence of the symptoms and the anatomic defect. As a result, some women with severe problems may have to modify their exercise habits appreciably.

Many women with minor problems, especially those with normal anatomy, may be able to control leakage by avoiding fluid ingestion for three hours prior to exercising and emptying their bladders immediately prior to exercising. However, they must be careful to avoid dehydration during prolonged exercise sessions lasting more than 1 hour, especially in hot weather. Such women should replace fluid loss immediately after cessation of exercise and should drink very small quantities during the exercise session.

Kegel exercises may also benefit many women who experience stress urinary incontinence. These are practiced by contracting the pubococcygeus muscle at any time, or specifically during urination, thereby interrupting the flow of urine. Wearing a minipad or panty liner is also helpful for many of those women who experience stress incontinence during exercise. Those who have anatomic abnormalities and are unable to relieve their symptoms sufficiently by practicing Kegel exercises or wearing a minipad should consider surgical repair of the defect. As mentioned above, such women may be at increased risk of postoperative recurrences as a result of pressure changes during exercise and persistence of the endogenous tissue factors that caused the original problem. Although no scientific data exist to confirm or refute this suspicion, these women should be cautious when exercising postoperatively.

Recommended Guidelines

All women should be encouraged to exercise regularly. Those who have already established the exercise habit should be encouraged to continue in programs that include regular aerobic exercise and strength training. As long as these women are healthy, are exercising properly, and are experiencing no problems with their programs, no changes are warranted. They should have the routine health screenings indicated for all women of the same age; no additional testing is indicated for their exercise.

For those women who have not begun to exercise regularly, especially those over age 40, a complete history and thorough physical examination are necessary, looking for specific symptoms suggestive of underlying cardiovascular disease (chest pain, dizziness, dyspnea on exertion, and so on). Although tests are not helpful in detecting disease in the asymptomatic patient, symptomatic patients should be evaluated by a cardiologist prior to initiating an exercise program. It is likely that this assessment will include an exercise electrocardiogram, or "stress test." For those women who have physical restrictions due to medical or musculoskeletal conditions, exercise programs must be carefully and individually planned to include only activities that can be performed safely and comfortably and to exclude any that are dangerous or uncomfortable.

Aerobic Exercise

Healthy women should be encouraged to engage in regular aerobic exercise for at least 30 minutes per session and repeated at least 3 times each week. The exercise should be intense enough to raise the heart rate to at least 100 beats per minute, and the intensity may be judged by perception of effort, rather than by actually measuring the heart rate. This goal can be achieved by any exercise that involves continual movement of large muscle groups without interruption, such as running, brisk walking, bicycling, aerobic dancing, rowing, or swimming. Women can be instructed in the basic principles so that they can modify their programs as needed. For example, some women prefer to combine different sports into one session in order to carry out the intended exercise without straining aging muscles, tendons, and joints. Some may find water exercises more comfortable since these will avoid the forces and impacts incurred by running on the ground.

Strength Training

Healthy women should be encouraged to practice weight training 2 or 3 times each week, using either resistance machines or free weights and exercising several different muscle groups for maximum benefit. They should be instructed in proper technique and should be supervised until it has been determined that they have mastered the technique and routine. After this level of competency has been attained, exercise may be continued safely without supervision.

Flexibility

A program of stretching exercises should be recommended for exercisers as well as sedentary women. Both intense exercise and aging contribute to a progressive shortening of muscle fibers, thereby reducing flexibility and limiting the ability to perform many specific exercises. Thus muscles should be stretched, preferably when they have been warmed by exercising, in order to maintain their elasticity and flexibility.

Compliance

In order to ensure that the prescribed exercise program can be followed, it is important to review with each woman her personal daily schedule to ensure that the planned program can be accommodated. It is unrealistic to assume that exercise will be added to a schedule that is already full, unless the woman is convinced that this exercise program is more important than some other activities, which will have to be eliminated to permit time for the exercise. Thus, it is important to take the necessary time to explain the benefits of exercise and the principles of the prescribed program. Several visits, in close temporal proximity to the initial exercise prescription, will be very helpful in confirming compliance, answering questions that have arisen, and monitoring progress and problems. Once the first 3 months of this new program have passed, and as long as the program seems to be progressing satisfactorily, routine annual visits will be sufficient. Such early program monitoring is essential to avoid most cases of early attrition.

Hormone Replacement Therapy

Hormone replacement therapy (HRT) refers to combined therapy with estrogen and progesterone (or a synthetic progestin). Estrogen replacement therapy (ERT) refers to therapy with estrogen alone. Estrogen is often prescribed to prevent osteoporosis and cardiovascular disease and to relieve vasomotor and urogenital symptoms. Progesterone (or a synthetic progestin) is added to the estrogen therapy only to protect the endometrium from the stimulating effects of unopposed estrogen. Thus any woman who has no uterus should not add progesterone (or a synthetic progestin) to her estrogen therapy schedule.

Benefits of Hormone Replacement Therapy

Cardiovascular Effects   Estrogen helps reduce cardiovascular risks by raising HDL cholesterol levels and lowering LDL cholesterol levels. Estrogen also has a favorable effect on blood vessel walls and blood flow. It remains to be shown how the effects of estrogen compare with those of exercise upon cardiovascular disease risks and whether the combination of estrogen supplementation and regular exercise provides greater benefit than either one alone.

Bone Effects   Estrogen has a beneficial effect on bone as well, and this also occurs by several mechanisms. Estrogen increases intestinal absorption of calcium and decreases bone resorption of calcium. We know from data collected in younger amenorrheic athletes that exercise alone cannot prevent osteopenia in hypoestrogenic amenorrheic athletes. Low body weight and inadequate calcium intake are common among such athletes and serve as confounding variables. We also know that calcium supplementation does not prevent bone loss as well as estrogen does. Most studies of estrogen therapy, calcium supplementation, and exercise have suffered from variable compliance and group overlap, thereby making it difficult to draw valid conclusions about the relative effects of these three factors. However, conclusions from published data indicate that 1) the combination of estrogen therapy, calcium supplementation, and exercise is more beneficial than any one or two of these, and 2) estrogen therapy is more effective in preserving bone density than exercise, calcium, or both (see Figure 13.1 and Tables 13.1 and 13.2).

Vasomotor Symptoms   Estrogen is the most effective treatment for vasomotor symptoms. No other therapy approaches estrogen in effectiveness.

Urogenital Atrophy   Estrogen is the most effective treatment for symptoms of urogenital atrophy.

Depression and Other Mood Disorders   Some forms of depression occur perimenopausally and postmenopausally. Although depression is often a complex and multifactorial disorder, a subset of depressed patients have menopause as an etiology. Because many menopausal women experience vasomotor symptoms and sleep disturbances that lead to chronic sleep deprivation, mood disorders and depression are sometimes seen in this group of women as a result. Estrogen therapy is the most effective way to improve sleep quality in these women, and it usually relieves the depression or other mood disturbances, as long as they resulted from sleep deprivation due to menopausal hormonal changes. Estrogen will not relieve depression that is caused by other factors that require psychotropic medication and appropriate counseling instead. It is unfortunate that

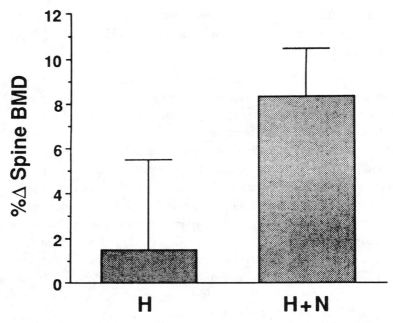

Figure 13.1 *Percentage change (mean ± SEM) in the BMD of surgical menopausal women after 1 year hormone therapy alone or hormone therapy plus Nautilus exercise. The probability (one-tailed t-test) associated with the change in spine BMD measures within the estrogen + exercise group (H + N) was* p = 0.002. *The probability (one-tailed t-test) associated with the change in spine BMD measures within the hormone-only group (H) was* p = 0.44. *Changes between groups were not significant. (Reproduced by permission from Notelovitz M, Martin D, Tesar R, et al. Estrogen therapy and variable-resistance weight training increase bone mineral in surgically menopausal women. J Bone Min Res 1991;6:583–590.)*

most women who experience this problem are often hopeful that only estrogen is necessary to correct the disturbance, and many of them are less willing to consult a psychiatrist than a gynecologist for advice. Optimally, a mental health specialist should be involved in the treatment plan for all such women.

Risks of Hormone Replacement Therapy

Endometrium   Unopposed estrogen (estrogen without progestin) imparts a risk of endometrial hyperplasia and adenocarcinoma and should not be

Table 13.1 *Dietary sources of calcium*

Food	Portion Size	Calcium (mgm)	Calories
Skim milk	8 oz.	250	90
Whole milk	8 oz.	250	160
Yogurt (low-fat fruit-flavored)	8 oz.	250	260
Cheddar cheese	1 oz.	250	100
Swiss cheese	1 oz.	250	100
Cottage cheese	10 oz.	250	300
Sardines with bones	3 oz.	250	300
Spinach, fresh or frozen	10 oz.	250	75

Reproduced by permission from Shangold M, Mirkin G. Older women. In: Shangold M, Mirkin G. The complete sports medicine book for women, Revised Edition. New York: Fireside 1992, p. 160.

prescribed to any woman who has a uterus. Rare exceptions to this recommendation exist; such women must be carefully monitored with frequent endometrial biopsies.

Breast The long-term effects of ERT and HRT on breast cancer risk remain controversial. Most studies have demonstrated no effect from HRT on the risk of developing breast cancer. However, a few studies have reported a slight increase in risk, and these studies have received much more publicity, especially in the lay press. Careful review of these studies leads to the conclusion that any increase in breast cancer risk, if it exists, must be quite small and may result from the method of reporting the data. The most appropriate conclusion to be drawn from the literature on this subject seems to be that HRT does not affect a woman's risk of developing breast cancer.

Coagulation Most forms of estrogen affect coagulation factors in ways that promote hypercoagulation. Thus women at risk for these problems should be monitored carefully.

Contraindications to Hormone Replacement Therapy

Women should not be treated with HRT if they have abnormal liver function, since estrogen and progestins are metabolized in the liver. Those

Table 13.2 *Elemental calcium in over-the-counter products*

Supplement	Amount of Elemental Calcium (mg)	Manufacturer
Calcium carbonate (40% calcium)		
Caltrate 600	600.0	Lederle
Calciday 667 mg	266.8	Nature's Bounty
Os-Cal 500 mg	500.0	Marion Merrell Dow
Ost-Cal 500 mg	500.0	Goldline
Ostercal 500 mg	500.0	Nature's Bounty
Oyster Shell Calcium 500 mg	500.0	Vangard
Rolaids Calcium Rich 550 mg	220.0	Warner-Lambert
Tums 500 mg	200.0	Norcliff Thayer
Tums E-X Extra Strength 750 mg	300.0	Norcliff Thayer
Calcium Citrate (21% calcium)		
Citracal 950 mg	200.0	Mission
Calcium lactate (14% calcium)		
Calcium lactate	42.25	Dixon-Shane, Geneva Marsam, Rugby
Calcium gluconate (9% calcium)		
Calcium gluconate		
500 mg	45.0	Dixon-Shane,
650 mg	58.5	Genetco, Lannett,
975 mg	87.75	Eli Lilly, Major,
1000 mg	90.0	Roxane, Rugby, Schein, URL, West-Ward

Source: Adapted from: Facts and comparisons, Philadelphia: JB Lippincott, 1991.

who have a previous thrombotic or embolic event must be evaluated very carefully to determine the etiology of that event before HRT can be prescribed safely. HRT should not be prescribed to any woman who has had breast cancer or endometrial cancer, with very rare exceptions, all of whom must be determined on an individualized basis. (Endometrial cancer is an absolute contraindication, except for those with early Stage I lesions, following definitive treatment. Breast cancer is also an absolute contraindication, but some women who have been treated more than 5 or 10 years previously and who have apparently been successfully treated and cured may be treated with HRT for significant improvement in their quality of life.) Any woman with undiagnosed vaginal bleeding should not be treated with HRT until a diagnosis has been established and the condition has been treated.

Other contraindications are relative, including migraine headaches, uterine myomata, and benign breast disease. Each of these needs to be evaluated individually, and the therapeutic plan needs to be determined on a case-by-case basis.

Prescribing Regimens

Older therapeutic regimens were based on the calendar month and were intended to simulate the hormonal events of a natural cycle in a premenopausal woman. Women were usually treated with estrogen for the first 25 days of the calendar month; a progestin was added on the last 7 to 10 days of estrogen for endometrial protection. When it was learned that 12 days of progestin therapy provided better endometrial protection than only 7 or 10 days, the standard prescribing regimen was modified to include progestin on the last 12 days of estrogen therapy. This regimen consisted of a progestin given on days 14 to 25 of every calendar month. If bleeding occurred, it usually did so at a predictable time: at or near the end of progestin therapy. No bleeding or bleeding at this time was medically acceptable; bleeding at any other time warranted evaluation.

Prescribing regimens were changed to eliminate the hormone-free days at the end of each calendar month because many women experienced a recurrence of symptoms at that time and because the 25-day schedule was actually dissimilar to the natural menstrual cycle that treatment sought to simulate. This change led to the prescribing of daily estrogen (skipping no days at the end of each calendar month). Based on a monthly cycle of hormone ingestion, women were instructed to begin the 12-day course of progestin on the first of the month, since the first of the month was an easier and more convenient starting date. In this schedule too, no bleeding

or bleeding at or near the end of progestin therapy was medically acceptable; bleeding at any other time required evaluation.

Shortly afterward, combined continuous hormonal therapy was intro-
duced, in which the woman takes both estrogen and progestin every day.
This prescribing regimen was intended to produce an atrophic endometrium from which no bleeding would take place. One of the major
disadvantages of this plan is a very high incidence of irregular and
unpredictable bleeding for the first 4 to 6 months, by which time endometrial atrophy is usually achieved. This prescribing regimen involves a
lower daily dose of progestin than is prescribed during cyclic therapy,
thereby reducing the likelihood of undesirable side effects and metabolic
effects from the progestational agent.

Although many women are taking combined continuous hormonal
therapy and are pleased to have no side effects and no vaginal bleeding,
many women prefer to have bleeding occur at a predictable time and
are more comfortable taking cyclic progestational therapy. Some of

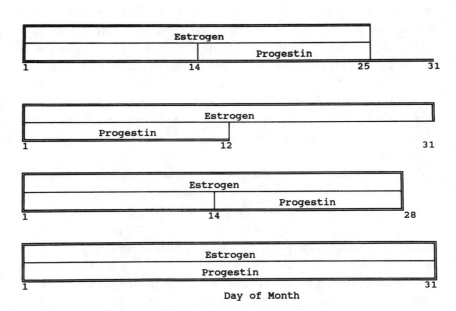

Figure 13.2   *HRT prescribing schedules*

Table 13.3 *Recommended prevention of and treatment for menopausal problems*

Vasomotor symptoms	Estrogen
Urogenital atrophy	Estrogen
Osteoporosis	Estrogen, calcium, exercise
Cardiovascular disease	Estrogen, exercise, low-fat diet
Obesity	Exercise
Depression and sleep disturbances	Estrogen, exercise, psychotropic medication, counseling

these women take 12 days of progestin, beginning on the first day of each calendar month. Others follow a 28-day cycle, in which estrogen is taken alone for 14 or 16 days, and this is followed by both estrogen and progestin for the remaining 14 or 12 days of the 28-day cycle. A new 28-day cycle is initiated as soon as the preceding one is completed (see Figure 13.2).

Side effects of estrogen include nausea, edema, mastalgia, breast enlargement, weight gain, headaches, growth of uterine myomata, vaginal bleeding, and predisposition to vaginal yeast infections. Side effects of progesterone and synthetic progestins include acne, skin oiliness, weight gain, mood changes, depression, lethargy, and vaginal bleeding. Dosages and prescribing schedules can usually be modified to eliminate or at least minimize these side effects (see Table 13.3).

Summary

The major symptoms and problems experienced by peri- and postmenopausal women are vasomotor symptoms, urogenital atrophy, cardiovascular disease, bone loss, muscle weakness, depression and sleep disturbances, and weight gain. Regular exercise will have a beneficial effect on cardiovascular disease risk, bone loss, muscle weakness, certain types of depression and sleep disturbances, and weight gain. HRT will have a beneficial effect on vasomotor symptoms, urogenital atrophy, cardiovascular disease risk, bone loss, and certain types of depression and sleep disturbances. Thus, all menopausal women should be encouraged to exercise regularly, and most will benefit from HRT unless contraindicated.

Bibliography

1. Åstrand I. Aerobic work capacity in men and women with special reference to age. Acta Physiol (Scand) 1960;49:1–92.

2. Blair SH, Kohl HW III, Paffenbarger RS, et al. Physical fitness and all-cause mortality: a prospective study of healthy men and women. JAMA 1989; 262:2395–2401.

3. Bogardus C, Lillioja S, Ravussin E, et al. Familial dependence of the resting metabolic rate. N Engl J Med 1986;315:96–100.

4. Caramelli KE, Notelovitz M. Effect of load-bearing during treadmill walking in women aged 57 to 67 years. Maturitas 1984;6:95. Abstract.

5. Cavanaugh DJ, Cann DE. Brisk walking does not stop bone loss in post menopausal women. Bone 1988;9:201–204.

6. Cohn SH, Abesamis C, Ysaumura S, et al. Comparative skeletal mass and radial bone mineral content in black and white women. Metabolism 1977;26:171–178.

7. Cowan MM, Gregory LW. Responses of pre- and postmenopausal females to aerobic conditioning. Med Sci Sports Exerc 1985;17:138–143.

8. Cunningham DA, Hill JS. Effect of training on cardiovascular response to exercise in women. J Appl Physiol 1975;39:891–895.

9. DeLorme TL, Watkins AL. Technics of progressive resistance exercise. Arch Phys Med 1948;29:263–273.

10. Despres JP, Bouchard C, Savard R, et al. The effect of a 20-week endurance training program on adipose tissue morphology and lipolysis in men and women. Metabolism 1984;33:235–239.

11. Despres JP, Tremblay, A, Nadeau A, Bouchard C. Physical training and changes in regional adipose tissue distribution. Acta Med Scand 1988; 723(suppl):205–212.

12. Drinkwater B, Horvath S, Wells C. Aerobic power of females ages 10 to 69. J Gerontol 1975;30:385–394.

13. Franklin B, Buskirk E, Hodgson J, et al. Effects of physical conditioning on cardiorespiratory function, body composition, and serum lipids in relatively normal weight and obese middle-aged women. Int J Obes 1979;3:97–109.

14. Grimby G, Saltin B. The aging muscle. Clin Physiol 1983;3:209–218.

15. Hammar M, Berg G, Lindgren R. Does physical exercise influence the frequency of postmenopausal flushes? Acta Obstet Gynecol Scand 1990; 69:409–412.

16. Harting GH, Moore CE, Mitchell R, et al. Relationship of menopausal status and exercise level to HDL cholesterol in women. Exp Aging Res 1984;10:13–18.

17. Heikkinen J, Kurttila-Matero E, Kyllonen E, et al. Moderate exercise does not enhance the positive effect of estrogen on bone mineral density in postmenopausal women. Calif Tissue Int 1991;49(suppl):S83–S84.

18. Kirk S, Sharp CF, Elbaum N, et al. Effect of long-distance running on bone mass in women. J Bone Min Res 1989;4:515–522.

19. Krolner B, Toft B, Nielsen SP, Tondevold E. Physical exercise as prophylaxis against involutional vertebral bone loss: a controlled trial. Clin Sci 1983;64:541–546.

20. Lapidus L, Bengtsson C, Larsson B, et al. Distribution of adipose tissue and risk of cardiovascular disease and death: a 12-year follow-up of participants in the population study of women in Gothenburg, Sweden. Br Med J [Clin Res] 1984;289:1257–1261.

21. Leon AS, Connett J, Jacobs DR, Rauramaa R. Leisure-time activity levels and risk of coronary heart disease and death. The multiple risk factor intervention trial. JAMA 1987;259:2388–2395.

22. Meredith CN, Zackin MJ, Frontera WR, Evans WJ. Body composition and aerobic capacity in young and middle-aged endurance-trained men. Med Sci Sports Exerc 1987;19:557–563.

23. Mole PA, Stern JS, Schultz CL, et al. Exercise reverses depressed metabolic rate produced by severe caloric restriction. Med Sci Sports Exerc 1989;21:29–33.

24. Moore CE, Hartung GH, Mitchell RE, et al. The relationship of exercise and diet on high-density lipoprotein cholesterol levels in women. Metabolism 1983;32:189–196.

25. Notelovitz M, Martin D, Tesar R, et al. Estrogen therapy and variable-resistance weight training increase bone mineral in surgically menopausal women. J Bone Min Res 1991;6:583–590.

26. Orwoll ES, Ferar J, Oviatt SK, et al. The relationship of swimming exercise to bone mass in men and women. Arch Intern Med 1989;149:2197–2200.

27. Osteoporosis and activity. Lancet 1983;2:1365. Editorial.

28. Paffenbarger RS, Hyde RT, Wing AL, et al. A natural history of athleticism on cardiovascular health. JAMA 1984;252:491–495.

29. Plowman S, Drinkwater B, Horvath S. Age and aerobic power in women: a longitudinal study. J Gerontol 1979;34:512–520.

30. Pocock NA, Eisman JA, Yeates MG, et al. Physical fitness is a major determinant of femoral neck and lumbar spine bone mineral density. J Clin Invest 1986;78:618–621.

31. Pollock ML. How much exercise is enough? Physician Sportsmed 1978;6:50–64.
32. Probart CK, Notelovitz M, Martin D, et al. The effect of moderate aerobic exercise on physical fitness among women 70 years and older. Maturitas 1991;14:49–56.
33. Riggs BL, Wahner HW, Dunn WL, et al. Differential changes in bone mineral density of appendicular and axial skeleton with aging: relationship to spinal osteoporosis. J Clin Invest 1981;67:328–335.
34. Rookus MA, Rokebrand P, Burema J, Deurenberg P. The effect of pregnancy on the body mass index 9 months postpartum in 49 women. Int J Obes 1987;11:609–618.
35. Shimokata H, Tobin JD, Muller DC, et al. Studies in the distribution of body fat: I. Effects of age, sex, and obesity. J Gerontol 1989;44:M66–M73.
36. Sidney K, Shephard R. Frequency and intensity of exercise training for elderly subjects. Med Sci Sports Exerc 1978;10:125–131.
37. Simkin A, Ayalon J, Leichter I. Increased trabecular bone density due to bone-loading exercises in postmenopausal osteoporotic women. Calcif Tissue Int 1987;40:59–63.
38. Smith EL, Reddan W, Smith PE. Physical activity and calcium modalities for bone mineral increase in aged women. Med Sci Sports Exerc 1981;13:60–64.
39. Tremblay A, Despres JP, Leblanc C, Bouchard C. Sex dimorphism in fat loss in response to exercise-training. J Obes Weight Regul 1984;3:193–203.
40. Van Dam S, Gillespy M, Notelovitz M, Martin AD. Effect of exercise on glucose metabolism in postmenopausal women. Am J Obstet Gynecol 1988;159:82–86.
41. White MK, Yenter RA, Martin RB, et al. Effects of aerobic dancing and walking on cardiovascular function and muscular strength in postmenopausal women. J Sports Med 1984;24:159–166.
42. Wilmore JH. Alterations in strength, body composition, and anthropometric measurements consequent to a 10-week weight training program. Med Sci Sports Exerc 1974;6:133–138.
43. Zauner C, Notelovitz M, Fields CD, et al. Cardiorespiratory efficiency at submaximal work in young and middle-aged women. Am J Obstet Gynecol 1984;150:712–715.

Index

Ideal body weight, infertility and, 75, 76
Immune system, 94, 96
Incontinence, urinary, 5–6, 69–71
  menopausal, 147–148
Infarction, myocardial, 146
Infertility, 73–77
Injectable steroids, 89, 91
Injury
  exercise frequency and duration and, 141
  pregnancy and, 126
Inositol, 90
Insulin, pregnancy and, 116
Intra-abdominal pressure, stress urinary incontinence and, 148
Iron deficiency, 20

Joint alteration in pregnancy, 118

Kegel exercise, 70, 148
Ketones, 116

Laboratory testing in pubertal delay, 19
Lanolin, 89
Lasix; *see* Furosemide
LDL; *see* Low-density lipoproteins
Lean body mass, aging and, 143
Legislation
  anabolic steroids and, 95
  growth hormone use and, 101
  increased exercising by female and, 2
Levodopa, 90
LH; *see* Luteinizing hormone
Libido, steroid use and, 92
Lidocaine, 90
Lipid synthesis during pregnancy, 116
Liver function
  anabolic steroids and, 93–94, 95
  hormone replacement therapy and, 153–154
Low body weight
  in athletic discipline options and problems, 5
  menstrual dysfunction and, 6, 36
  in pubertal delay, 13, 15–18, 21–23
Low-density lipoproteins
  aerobic exercise and, 140
  hormone replacement therapy and, 150

steroid use and, 95
Luteal phase of menstrual cycle, 27, 28
  athletic performance and, 106, 108
  dysfunction, 31–34, 39
    infertility and, 75
    management, 44
    menopause and, 138
Luteinizing hormone, 29
  anorexia nervosa and, 41–42
  concentration of in swimmers, 38
  for infertility, 77
  in menstrual cycle, 26, 27, 28
  in menstrual dysfunction, 31, 32, 33, 39
Luteinizing hormone/follicle-stimulating hormone ratio
  infertility and, 76
  in menstrual dysfunction, 18
  swimming and, 18, 38
Lysine for growth hormone release, 99

Magnetic resonance imaging in pubertal delay, 19
Male hormone, 10, 11
Male pattern baldness, 93, 95
Masculinization
  anabolic steroid use and, 20
  menstrual dysfunction and, 39
Meat consumption, 64
Media, increased exercising by female and, 2
Medroxyprogesterone, 23, 44
Menarche, 10
  delayed; *see* Amenorrhea
  dysmenorrhea and, 52
  fractures and, 78
  growth spurt prior to, 11–12
  normal, 9–12
Menopause, 137–160
  exercise and, 137–140
    benefits, 140–145
    recommendations, 148–150
    risks, 146–147
  hormone replacement therapy, 150–157
Menses, 27
Menstrual cycle
  athletic performance and, 106–108
  dysfunction; *see* Amenorrhea; Menstrual dysfunction
  initiation; *see* Menarche